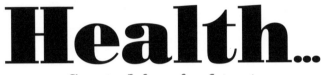

Health...

Great advice, simply put

Health...

Great advice, simply put

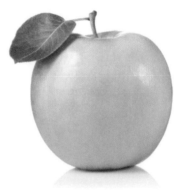

Easy ways to feel better and live longer

Joe Kita
and the staff of READER'S DIGEST magazine

Published by The Reader's Digest Association, Inc.
London • New York • Sydney • Montreal

FOR VIVAT DIRECT
Editorial Director Julian Browne
Art Director Anne-Marie Bulat
Managing Editor Nina Hathway
Trade Books Editor Penny Craig
Picture Resource Manager Eleanor Ashfield
Prepress Technical Manager Dean Russell
Production Controller Jan Bucil
Product Production Manager Claudette Bramble

Book code 400-608
ISBN 978 1 78020 136 8

Printing and binding Arvato Iberia, Portugal

'I don't want to get to the end of my life and find that I just lived the length of it. I want to have lived the width of it as well.'

DIANE ACKERMAN, *AUTHOR*

'When it comes to eating right and exercising, there is no 'I'll start tomorrow.' Tomorrow is disease.'

TERRI GUILLEMETS, *ANTHOLOGIST*

'The greatest wealth is health.'

VIRGIL, *ROMAN POET*

'If you break a leg, don't come running to me.'

CONNIE KITA, *THE AUTHOR'S MOTHER*

Contents

INTRODUCTION

When I was a boy, Dr Rutledge was our family doctor. His surgery was a small brick building, with a wondrous aquarium in the waiting room that made it seem as if you were never waiting very long. He worked in shirt-sleeves without gloves and smelled like Clubman hair tonic. His receptionists greeted us by name with genuine smiles, and I can't remember Dr Rutledge ever making a referral; he just seemed to fix everything right there in the surgery. And when your diagnosis was complete, he personally presented you – whether child or adult – with a lollipop.

Now, some forty years later, my family sees a raft of different health practitioners, even though we're all healthy. Today you

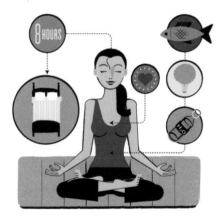

are lucky if you see the same doctor twice for the same health problem, a nurse comes from the local hospital to do blood tests and you see a practice nurse to get your blood pressure checked. The waiting rooms of today's multi-doctor practices are all unadorned and the wait is interminable. We're recognised by our files, not our faces. And the receptionist's first words are always, 'What's your date of birth?'

Should one of us ever get really sick and have to 'negotiate' the health system, we'll probably need to be our own advocates because things are so complex. And lollipops? Well, those spike blood sugar and promote obesity, you know.

Having been a health journalist for 30 years, I worry that patients are losing their patience. Most people nowadays are so overwhelmed by the medical system and its seemingly endless reorganisations, not to mention the bombardment of so much contradictory health and nutrition information by the media,

Staying healthy shouldn't cause you stress. Here is simple, empowering advice for making health easy – even pleasurable – to maintain.

that they're at the brink of inaction. Staying healthy has become a source of stress rather than satisfaction.

That's why *Reader's Digest* has decided to do what it does best – gather and condense the most vital information on the topic of health and present it in a way that educates, enlightens and empowers you. Although not in any way designed to replace professional medical care, it is intended to simplify it. On the following pages, you'll find succinct, practical, straightforward advice on 70 essential facets of health, fitness, nutrition, and overall well-being. From snoring to skin cancer, cholesterol to cold sores, weight loss to waiting times... it's all here.

So turn the page and step into *our* office. The people are friendly, you won't be told there are no appointments available this week and there's no waiting. And although we couldn't include a lollipop in the package, we guarantee you'll leave feeling this is one challenge you have unquestionably licked.

JOE KITA

Living well...

Instead of viewing life as a discount store, where quantity is the driving force, it's time to start looking at it as a smaller, more specialist shop, where quality is paramount. As evidenced at nursing homes nationwide, it's not the number of days in your life that matters but the amount of life in those days. All the advice in this section – from lowering stress to boosting energy to making love last – is designed to do just that. If living well is an art, consider this your foundation course.

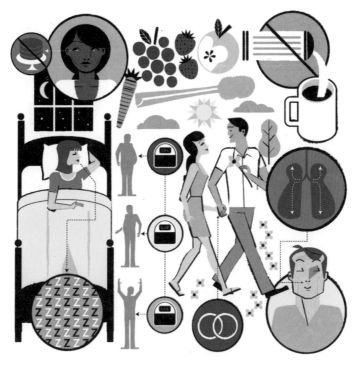

Sleep well
tonight (and every night)

If doctors took the time to pinpoint the cause of disease, the words 'lack of sleep' would appear on many death certificates. Heart disease, stroke, diabetes, obesity, depression, even cancer are linked to not getting adequate rest – something of which more than 50 per cent of Britains are guilty. Experts now estimate that the significantly sleep-deprived have a poorer quality of life and a 20 per cent greater risk of death than the well rested. If you're tossing and turning, here's how to finally rest easy.

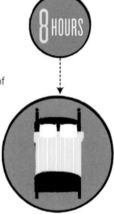

Calculate and commit
For every two hours of wakefulness, you need one hour of sleep. So if you're up for 16 hours, you should be down for eight. Do the maths, and remember that sleep debt is cumulative. If you're not meeting your quota during the week, catch up on the weekend. Once you know how much rest you require, prioritise it. Sleeping is not a sign of laziness; it's the simplest, most important thing you can do for better health.

Set a caffeine deadline
This should generally be 10 hours before bedtime. Caffeine has a half-life of about six hours, which means that 50 per cent of what's ingested at noon is in your system at 6 P.M., and half of that still lingers at midnight. So the earlier you have your last hit, the better. And this includes caffeinated teas, fizzy drinks, even chocolate.

Exercise regularly

Thirty minutes of moderate daily exercise produces feel-good hormones called endorphins that promote and deepen sleep. (Just avoid exercising within three hours of bedtime.)

Eat early and light

Allow four hours for digestion prior to bed, and make dinner the lightest meal of the day. Likewise, have your nightcap three hours before bed in order to give your body time to metabolise the alcohol.

> **LIVING UNDER THE INFLUENCE**
>
> » After 17 to 19 hours without sleep, your brain activity is similar to someone with a blood alcohol content of 50 mg per 100ml of blood. (The legal limit for drink-driving in the UK is 80 mg.)

Prepare the bat cave

Your bedroom should be dark, cool and quiet. Block all ambient light, including the illuminated face of your alarm clock (turn it towards the wall). Make sure you're warm enough and use cotton pyjamas and sheets. Keep TVs and computers out of the bedroom, and mask any outside noise with the continuous low hum of a fan or a radio set between stations.

Flush

When you go to the bathroom for the final time, spend a few extra minutes writing your worries on a piece of tissue. Then throw it in the bowl and flush. There now, your mind is clear. Pleasant dreams...

Lose weight
for good

The reason most diets fail is because they require us to give up the foods we love. Still, we vow to be strong, bravely resist for weeks and then, in a moment of weakness, we succumb to a craving, our diet disintegrates and eventually we rebound to an even higher weight. If this sounds familiar, you should know there's a way to break this cycle and lose weight for good *without* swearing off your favourite foods.

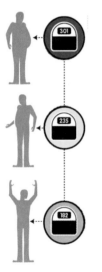

Rather than changing *what* you eat, the secret is changing *how* you eat it. To lose weight, simply eat from a smaller plate, researchers say. The size of plate we use makes a big difference a study in the US found. These ideas might seem trivial, but by eating a little less at every meal, you will steadily return to your more natural weight.

Switch from dinner to salad plates

Researchers at Cornell University in the US found that switching from 26cm to 20cm plates (and, of course, not indulging in seconds) reduced calorie consumption by about 20 per cent per meal. Not only does a smaller-diameter plate hold less food, it also creates an illusion of plenty by appearing full. This tricks the mind into feeling satisfied with less food.

Choose smaller bowls

In another study people who served themselves ice cream in 500g bowls ate 31 per cent less than those using bowls holding twice as much. And again, they didn't feel cheated, because the portion appeared relatively substantial.

Use a smaller scoop

The people in the study who served themselves with a 2oz ice-cream scoop ingested nearly 15 per cent less than those using 3oz scoops. When small bowls *and* small spoons were used, 57 per cent less ice cream was consumed without anyone feeling shortchanged. Eating with a smaller spoon might help, too. Since there's about a 20-minute lag between when your belly is full and the point at which your brain recognises it, slowing your eating with smaller utensils helps you savour food more, causing you to naturally bridge that gap and eat less.

Select a small glass

Using short, wide drinking glasses typically results in about 20 per cent less liquid being consumed compared to tall, skinny ones. Keep this in mind when drinking soft drinks and alcohol.

Run with this concept

The possibilities for downsizing your dinnerware (and yourself!) are endless. For instance, use smaller serving utensils in casserole dishes. Set out smaller knives to spread cream cheese and butter. Swirl pasta around a smaller fork. Cut your food into tinier pieces. Buy kid-size snack packages... To win the war on big, think small.

THE KEY QUESTION Before embarking on any diet, ask yourself: can I eat this way for the rest of my life? If the answer is no, then don't even start. Although subsisting on cabbage soup or mail-order diet meals may help you lose weight short-term, you'll inevitably tire of such restrictions. To be successful long-term, a diet shouldn't be a diet; it should be a lifestyle.

Avoid home
health traps

Y ou fret about catching the latest media-hyped disease
or whether your food is chemical-free, but one of the
biggest threats to your family's health is right under your roof.
More than one million children under the age of 15 are taken
to accident and emergency units following accidents in and
around the home every year. Instead of cleaning the toilets this
weekend, here are the five biggest threats to address.

Keeping everybody upright
Falls are a leading cause of home injury and death, especially
among children and older adults. So wipe out slipperiness in
your house. Secure shaky railings, put nonslip strips in the bath
and under rugs, keep stairs clear, install nightlights in bedroom
and bath areas, put guards or locks on toddlers' windows,
spread fresh mulch around play areas and replace those old
step stools and ladders Grandpa gave you.

Protecting against poisoning
Make sure you secure anything that can be accessed and
accidentally ingested by a child (medicines, vitamins, cleaning
liquids, your brother's home brew...). But pills and fluids aren't
the only potential poisons. Known as the silent killer, carbon
monoxide can be emitted from gas fires, boilers and other gas
appliances. As it is odourless and deadly, install CO detectors
near bedrooms and have gas appliances checked regularly.

Preventing fires and burns
Assuming all your fire extinguishers and smoke detectors
are working, here are two things to check that most people
overlook. Open and push down on your oven door. If the entire

Living well...

oven tips forward, call an appliance service to secure it. Next, inspect your boiler for signs of deterioration and leakage. It's one of the most dangerous appliances in the house and needs to be regularly maintained to prevent explosions. Check the temperature setting against the manufacturer's instructions.

Breathing easy

Dive into the kids' toy chest and do the toilet roll test. Anything small enough to fit through one is a choking hazard for children under five. Next, remove all pillows, blankets and toys from the baby's cot – these are suffocation risks, as is putting the little one to sleep on his chest or side. As for better air quality in your home, wage war on dust by sweeping often, use synthetic doormats (they don't get mouldy), keep an eye on bathroom mould and keep windows open as much as possible.

Staying afloat

Water holds a particular fascination for young children. Check your garden regularly. Containers holding rainwater should be emptied or sealed to prevent children gaining access, and paddling pools should always be emptied and turned upside down after use. If you have a pool or pond, ensure that it is inaccessible to a child who may escape supervision.

ARE YOU SMOKING WITHOUT REALISING IT? Smoking is the leading cause of lung cancer. No surprise there. But were you aware that radon, an odourless and invisible gas, is the runner-up? It's even more deadly than secondhand smoke. Radon comes from decaying uranium, which exists naturally in the earth in many parts of the world. It can work its way through home foundations and even into water. Visit hpa.org.uk to find out about home testing kits and learn more.

Brave a **craving**

Life is one big constant crave. Whether it's food, beauty, money, gadgets, sex or status, we are an incredibly rich society that somehow still needs everything. For proof, just look in your wardrobe, garage or rented storage unit. Or even more troubling, look at your middle in the mirror. In fact, let's start there. If you can learn to control your food cravings, which are the most frequent and irresistible of all, you'll be on your way to resisting other temptations as well.

Determine what you're really hungry for

The next time you get a craving, ask yourself if you're stressed, frustrated, sad or bored. If so, then you're eating to fill an emotional void rather than a physical one. Try keeping a 'desire diary' for a week. Whenever a craving strikes, note your mood. If stress turns out to be your trigger, exercise more to relieve the pressure. If it's loneliness that's driving you to the Doritos bag, call someone or join a social network such as Facebook or Meetup. Remember also that true hunger is easy to satisfy; any food will do. But emotional hunger usually manifests in desires for specific things like chocolate, ice cream or McDonald's.

Get off the energy roller coaster

The second biggest cause of cravings is a diet with too much refined carbohydrate. This causes drops in blood sugar that prompt hunger. For instance, if you have a chocolate croissant for breakfast, you'll get a nice jolt of energy from the sugar, but by mid-morning you'll be craving another. To stabilise energy

Living well...

levels and appetite, eat more protein and fibre. Tomorrow have eggs and wholemeal toast or a bowl of fibre-rich cereal with nuts and see if you can easily make it to lunch.

Stay hydrated

Many people think they're hungry when they're actually thirsty. To test if a food craving is genuine, drink a glass of water and wait a few minutes to see if it subsides. At the very least, you'll be better hydrated.

15» The number of minutes of walking it takes to successfully stifle a chocolate craving. Sceptical? Try it. If the urge doesn't subside, then indulge yourself. At least you'll already have burned a good chunk of the calories.

Distract yourself

Taste buds have a very short attention span. Instead of instantly giving in to a craving, have a mint, brush your teeth, check emails, call a friend or just wait five minutes. In most cases, you'll find you weren't really hungry.

Redo your kitchen

Put all your crave foods on the lowest or highest shelf in the back of the fridge or in the cupboard you need a stool to reach. This will give you more time to think before you eat.

Hang on to your hair

We all know that guys often lose their hair. But here's an interesting statistic: a man's age gives a good approximation of the probability that he has started balding. For example, at the age of 50, chances that you've started balding are around 50 per cent. Less known, and more frightening, is that about 55 per cent of women experience hair loss at some point in their lives. Often this starts during menopause. Although hair loss is mostly an inherited condition resulting from a complex gene interaction, there are some simple things you can do to avoid triggering it sooner and retain more of what you have for longer.

Save on products
Despite how Rihanna makes it seem when she dances, hair is not a living thing. Once it pops out of your head, it's dead. So for retention purposes, it's better to focus on what's happening below the surface, or inside the hair follicle. Most people think of it the other way around.

Learn to relax
Stress, whether it's ongoing anxiety from work or a traumatic event like the death of a friend, can prompt hereditary hair loss to start sooner – a condition called shedding. Manage your stress better by adopting a yoga mindset. Here's the mantra: *I can't control what happens, but I can control my reaction to what happens.* Just that little shift in thinking can make a big difference. Try it.

Stop dieting
Hair follicles, like all living organisms, need good nutrition to function. So don't starve yours by going on restrictive fad diets. The body interprets these as another form of stress. Instead,

Living well...

control weight with exercise and smarter eating. Vegetarians should make sure to meet RDAs for protein and iron, since deficiencies in either can cause hair loss. (Forget special hair vitamins, though; there's no clinical proof they work.)

Keep the blood flowing

Hair follicles also require good circulation to flourish. Regular aerobic exercise strengthens the heart so it can pump more blood up there. Likewise, keep your arteries lean and flexible by eating a low-fat, fibre-rich diet and not smoking.

DON'T WORRY, IT'S NORMAL

50 to 100 »

The average number of hairs per day the average person loses from his or her scalp.

Assess your meds

Certain medications and supplements can trigger hair loss. Among them are antidepressants, beta-blockers, steroids and even too much vitamin A. If you notice thinning after you start popping a new pill, check the side effects and discuss alternatives with your doctor.

Wear a hat

A bad sunburn on the scalp releases an inflammatory compound called superoxide that causes follicles to shut down. Contrary to popular belief, hats don't prompt hair loss; they protect against it.

Consult a hair doctor

If you're particularly worried, ask a dermatologist to assess the condition of your scalp and hair. Someone who specialises in skin and hair disorders will also look at possible medical treatment of the underlying cause. She can do a scalp biopsy to determine if it's temporary or longer lasting, and you can discuss regrowth options.

Be a smarter supermarket shopper

If your supermarket trips have become super-long because of all the label reading and brand comparison you're doing, it's time to streamline your strategy. Here are some quick ways to determine whether a product is healthy or hyped.

Forget about package claims

Terms such as 'natural', 'good source of...', 'low fat', and even 'whole grain' are all unregulated marketing buzzwords. A survey by consumer watchdog Which? found that food label claims such as 'pure', 'fresh', 'non-artificial', 'natural' and 'real' are largely unregulated and are confusing shoppers. For example, a product may be labelled 'made with real fruit juice' yet contain just a small amount. 'Lower fat' often merely means that a high-fat product has had the content trimmed a little, not that it is healthy.

Scan the ingredients

Nina Planck, a real-food expert and author, recommends paying more attention to a product's ingredient list than its nutrition facts panel. She contends that counting calories, grams of protein and other nutrients takes the enjoyment out of eating by making it a confusing science. Instead, when deciding between brands, she simply chooses the one with the fewest and most recognisable ingredients. Doing so usually guarantees she's buying food that's 'whole', or closer to its original state, and thus more healthy.

Beware these words

If, among the ingredients, you spot high-fructose corn syrup (or other words ending in 'ose', such as maltose, dextrose and sucrose), hydrogenated oils, artificial flavours and colours or anything you can't pronounce, put the item back on the shelf. Corn syrup and other added sugars have been linked to obesity and its many woes, while hydrogenated oils and chemical additives can promote cancers.

Check a few key facts

Two-thirds of shoppers read nutrition panels, but fewer than half understand them. So don't try to digest the whole thing. Instead, focus on three statistics: 1) saturated fat (should be less than 7 per cent of total daily value); 2) sodium (should be less than 300mg per serving); and 3) serving size (should not be so small that you can easily eat three or more at a sitting, which multiplies all values accordingly).

Shop naked

The best foods are those that don't come dressed in packages. Fresh fruits and vegetables, for example, don't need any hype or analysis, because they are what they are, plain and simple. Fill your basket with them.

LET YOUR PHONE MAKE THE CALL A growing number of mobile phone apps enable shoppers to scan a product's barcode and receive an instant health rating. Many are currently only available only in the US, but some, such as Food Scanner, Superfood and Good Shopping Guide, are available in the UK. Make sure, however, that the app you choose is not marketed or sponsored by a food manufacturer, which may make it biased.

Best 10 minute workout:
Sun salutations

I t's better to do a little exercise a lot rather than a lot of exercise a little. The second approach will injure you, while the first one – even if it's just 10 minutes per day – will eventually make you fit, slim and healthy. Yoga classes traditionally begin with a series of ten postures linked in a continuous flowing motion that elevates heart rate, boosts metabolism and stretches and strengthens just about every muscle in the body. It's called a Sun Salutation. Start your day with 10 minutes' worth and enjoy the benefits.

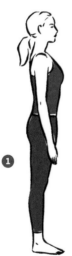

1. *Stand tall at the front of your mat with both feet touching and arms at your sides. Inhale and exhale deeply through the nose three times.*

2. *Inhale while extending and raising both arms overhead until palms meet. Gaze up.*

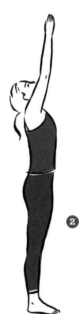

3. *Exhale and fold forward bringing your chest towards your knees and your head towards your toes. Hands should rest on the floor, ankles or knees.*

4. *Inhale and, without moving your hands, come up halfway, lengthening your spine and directing your gaze out in front.*

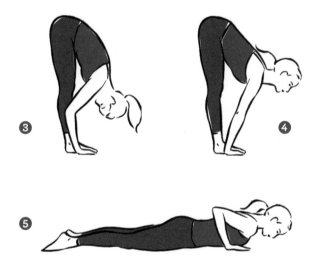

5. *Exhale and step back with one foot and then the other until you're in a high plank position. Keep elbows tucked, lower to the floor, as if finishing a push-up.*

6. *Inhale and straighten your arms while rolling on to the tops of your feet. Legs are extended behind as the chest approaches a 90-degree angle with the floor. This is called up-dog.*

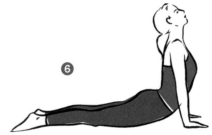

7. *Exhale and push back into down-dog. You should resemble an upside-down V, with fingers spread wide and heels on or pushing towards the floor. Let your head dangle. Hold the pose for five complete breaths.*

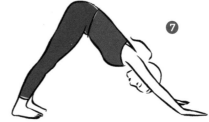

8. *Inhale while stepping one foot and then the other between your hands. Lengthen the spine and look ahead as in step 4.*

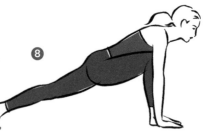

Living well...

9. *Exhale and fold forward as in step 3.*

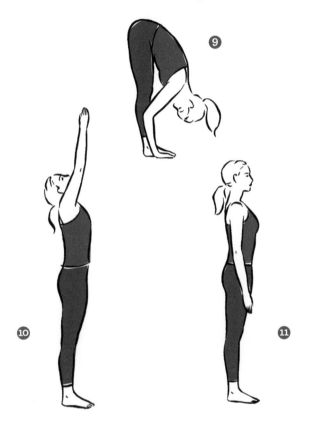

10. *Inhale while coming up and raising both arms as in step 2.*

11. *Lower arms back to the start position, take three breaths and repeat.*

Find your
ideal exercise

Exercise is the answer. When done regularly, it burns fat, brightens mood, fights disease and even makes you more attractive. So why don't more people embrace it? Because they haven't found the exercise they were designed for, both physically and psychologically. If your basement is a jungle of the latest advertised discarded gear, if you've quit more gyms than a pastry chef has eaten cupcakes, here's how to finally find your 'soul game'.

Match your personality
If you're an extrovert, then pedalling a stationary bike in your basement or watching exercise DVDs on your TV isn't going to satisfy you for long. Better to sign up for Zumba or join a team in training for a charity run or ride. Conversely, if you're a loner, then the solitary space that walking, running or a home gym affords should appeal to you more.

Match your body type
If you're naturally big-boned, then running and other high-impact activities will never be comfortable (or healthy) for you. Better to choose a weight-bearing exercise like spinning or swimming. Likewise, if you're smallish, then being in a weight room with a bunch of Amazonians will forever make you feel inferior. Try a more vigorous style of yoga, like Ashtanga, to tone your muscles.

Regress
To further hone in on your ideal exercise, think about the activities you enjoyed as a child. Maybe you loved skipping,

pedalling a bike or hiking and exploring in the woods. Revisit them. Chances are, even decades later you'll still experience the same joy.

Banish the word 'workout'

The power of suggestion is... well, powerful. Every time you refer to exercise as *working* out, you're creating a negative association in your subconscious. Instead, start thinking of it as playtime (mark it on your calendar as such) and see whether you anticipate it more.

Dabble

Many people find they have an ideal exercise *type* rather than just one perfect pastime. This is good. If you discover you feed off the energy of group classes, don't limit yourself to just one type or instructor. Change weekly or monthly. The variety will keep your mind and body fresh.

Consider one more alternative

Your ideal exercise may be much broader than you originally thought. Researchers are finding that being active throughout the day (housework, gardening, running errands) is better for overall well-being and even weight loss than confining activity to an hour or so and being sedentary the rest of the day. So if an exercise you try doesn't seem to click, just be more active.

GIVE IT THE TEST You'll know you've found your soul sport when the time you spend doing it becomes timeless. You'll look at your watch and be stunned an hour (or more!) has passed. This is known as flow, or being in the sweet spot. Relish it.

Beat fatigue,
boost energy

Ever wonder why zombies are so popular nowadays? We have a theory. Maybe it's because watching them stagger around makes us feel well rested by comparison. Indeed, we have become a Zombie Nation in ways beyond entertainment. A recent survey says one in three British workers suffers from poor sleep, and according to another survey by BUPA, the sleepless population is costing UK industry £1.6 billion a year, in lost productivity, accidents and illness. Here's how to leave the ranks of the living dead.

Pay off your sleep debt
Most people don't realise that sleep debt is cumulative. If you lose an hour or two a few nights in a row, you won't feel fresh until you make that down time up. Adults ideally need seven to nine hours of sleep per night, or 56 to 63 hours per week, to stay healthy and energised. Keep a weekly tally.

Become less chemically dependent
Resorting to caffeine, nicotine, alcohol or other stimulants to overcome fatigue is a short-term solution that can have debilitating long-term effects. Not only can you develop unhealthy dependencies on these substances, they can also interfere with sleep, which defeats the purpose of taking them in the first place.

Exercise to energise
Although it sounds contradictory, expending energy gives you *more* energy. This is due to the fatigue-fighting, mood-enhancing brain chemicals released during physical activity. Sceptical? Try this: the next time you need a pick-me-up, go for a walk or do some calisthenics. The exercise doesn't even have to be vigorous to make you feel more alert.

Living well...

Eat more often and more densely

Eating lots of unrefined carbohydrates, like white bread, rice and pasta, is akin to trying to keep a fire burning with newsprint. There's an immediate flare-up, but the flames subside quickly. Better to stoke yourself with a steady supply of denser, longer-burning, complex carbohydrate (whole grains, beans, fruits, vegetables) and lean protein. Even better, eat five or six smaller meals per day rather than the usual two or three. More frequent, more diverse eating will also supply a wider range of nutrients, which will help correct any deficiencies that may be compounding your tiredness.

Keep water in the tank

Being just 2 per cent underhydrated can make you act and feel older. For a sharp mind, smooth skin, better health and fluid movement, you need water. But forget about the old eight-times-eight rule (eight glasses of water daily). Healthy eaters, it turns out, get all the water they need from what they routinely eat and drink (that includes tea and coffee but not alcoholic beverages). If you're thirsty, though, drink up. And if you've worked up a sweat exercising, are in a hot climate or are taking medications, you may need to drink more than usual.

HAVE A NAP-A-LATTE TO GO There is nothing more naturally energy-boosting than a nap of 10 to 30 minutes. Dipping into just the first couple stages of sleep refreshes and restores alertness. Don't sleep any longer than that, though, or you'll awaken groggier than when you started, a condition called sleep inertia.

For those times when you need to power through, here's a recipe from sleep expert Michael Breus, PhD. He calls it a 'nap-a-latte': drink a lukewarm-to-cold cup of filter coffee (it has the most caffeine), then close your eyes for 20 to 25 minutes. 'You'll get just enough sleep to reduce fatigue, and when the caffeine kicks in, you'll be good for another four hours.'

Be your own
massage therapist

Studies show that regular massage is one of the simplest yet most effective ways to lower stress and boost mood. But it's an expensive habit if done by a pro, and most spouses will only indulge you after much begging and negotiating. So it's time to take matters into your own hands, so to speak. Here are our favourite self-massage tricks and techniques to finally get you rubbed the right way.

Let the good times roll
If you think of your muscles as dough that kneads to be relaxed, then you'll grasp the concept behind high-density foam rollers. Generally about 13cm thick and 30 to 91cm long, they're especially good for lying on and massaging a sore back or legs. For a cheaper alternative, try a swimming pool noodle, rolling pin or clean paint roller.

Smile constantly at work
Fill a self-seal bag with marbles and put it on the floor under your desk. Periodically remove your shoes and roll the stress away. (It's even more indulgent during long staff meetings.)

Slip into some new beans
Fill your slippers with a thin layer of small, uncooked beans and enjoy a foot massage while you clean. Bonus: if your spouse ticks you off by refusing to help, make chilli.

Turn the bathroom into a spa
Water massage is called hydrotherapy. If you have a whirlpool bath, position your lower back, the soles of your feet or any other aching muscle in front of a jet. Likewise, let the spray

from your showerhead gently massage your scalp, face, neck, back and shoulders.

Use the old sock-and-rice trick

If you haven't done this before, you're in for a treat. Find an old sports sock (but no holes!), fill it with rice, then securely tie the top. Put in the microwave and heat for 60 to 90 seconds. Lie the sock on any sore muscles for incredible relief as the rice contours to your body. It's particularly nice around the back of your neck. Don't empty the sock afterwards; use it over and over.

Have a ball

Just about any type of ball can be a self-massage tool. Roll a golf ball around with your toes, soothe sore shoulders and thighs with a cricket ball. Or stuff two tennis balls into a sock, tie the end and use the leverage from a floor or wall to roll them along your spine.

Train your pet to walk on your back

This works best with a small dog (as opposed to a canary or a Doberman). Lie facedown on the floor while a friend repeats a command such as 'Rubdown!' and uses a treat to entice the pet to walk around on your back. In time all you'll need to do is lie down, repeat the command and let Magic Paws take over. Cats also make great heating pads. Train yours to curl up on your back and you'll be purring in no time.

DONATE YOUR BODY TO SCIENCE If there's a school or further education college where they run massage courses near you, call to see if the students need any volunteer bodies to work on. You may be able to get a free massage or one for a good discount.

Decide if
organic is worth it

You know it's good for you, and you'd like to fill up your trolley with it. But if you're like most shoppers, you're probably aghast at the price of organic alternatives in the supermarket. If you're confused as to whether organic is worth the expense, here's some guidance.

Don't assume it's good for you

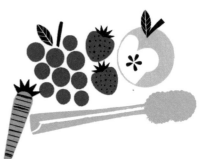

In the last few years 'organic' has become another marketing buzz word. As well as fruit and veg, there's now organic cake mix, sausages, ice cream, and even tobacco. It's an effective word, too. Many people believe, falsely, that products featuring the label are healthier, or lower in calories, than their non-organic counterparts. That's simply not true. So if you're out to lose weight and get fit, don't misinterpret eating organic as the way to do it.

Don't assume it's more nutritious

A large-scale study commissioned by the Food Standards Authority (FSA) found that there was no significant difference in vitamins and minerals between organic and standard food. What you're essentially buying when you choose organic is a pesticide- and chemical-free product that's better for the environment and less toxic for your body, not one with more vitamins and minerals.

Don't assume it tastes better

There's little research to support the notion that organic foods in general taste superior; any perceived difference is probably a case of justifying expense by using mind over platter. That said, *we* certainly think we taste the difference between locally grown produce bought the day after it was harvested and food raised on superfarms and shipped across the country. But that might have nothing to do with organics.

Clean up the largest part of your diet

If buying organic is important to you, there's no need to revamp your entire diet and blow your food budget. Many lower-priced, non-organic foods aren't much different from their organic counterparts. To help you decide which organics to buy, draw a food pyramid for your family. Put those things eaten most at the bottom and those consumed least up top. Then direct most of your organic food pounds at what's foundational. For instance, if you're a meat-eggs-and-potato family then buy organic in those areas, where it will have the most impact.

Know the lingo

All organic products are not created equal. The Food Standards Agency (FSA) states: 'Manufacturers of organic food are permitted to use specific non-organic ingredients provided that organic ingredients make up at least 95 per cent of the food.' If the product contains between 70 and 95 per cent organic ingredients, these can be mentioned only in the ingredients list, and a clear statement must be given on the front of the label showing the total percentage that are organic. Labels on food sold as 'organic' must also indicate the organic certification body that the producer of the food is registered with. The Soil Association Certification is the UK's largest organic certification body, and the one you're most likely to spot.

Grow your own

If you want superior taste and nutrition without the expense and confusion, plant an organic garden. Just-picked produce is the most healthy food of all, plus you'll have the added kudos of knowing you grew it.

WHEN TO SPEND, WHEN TO SAVE Each year the Government's Pesticide Residues Committee analyses pesticide residues on commercially sold produce. Generally, fruits contain more residue than vegetables because they are more prone to damage by pests. Here's our analysis of where to best spend your organic food pounds:

Buy Organic	Buy Regular
▶▶ Pears	▶▶ Cauliflower
▶▶ Bananas	▶▶ Sweetcorn
▶▶ Strawberries	▶▶ Broccoli
▶▶ Apricots	▶▶ Mushrooms
▶▶ Apples	▶▶ Courgettes
▶▶ Grapes	▶▶ Leeks
▶▶ Cherries	▶▶ Swede
▶▶ Raspberries	▶▶ Cabbage
▶▶ Melon	▶▶ Carrots
▶▶ Pineapples	▶▶ Asparagus
▶▶ Herbs	▶▶ Peppers
▶▶ Lettuce	▶▶ Avocado
▶▶ Celery	▶▶ Blueberries
▶▶ Potatoes	▶▶ Kiwi fruit

{ How can I live **more organically?** }

Live to 100+

It's not that difficult. The consensus of 100 doctors we polled is that at least 60 per cent of chronic disease can be avoided by doing 12 simple things. In fact, studies of identical twins, who share the same genes but not the same habits or environment, suggest DNA dictates only 25 to 33 per cent of life expectancy. But the following checklist isn't just a prescription for living long; it's your ticket to living well. And it's never too late to start.

1. **Stop smoking**
   Four years after doing so, your chance of having a heart attack falls to that of someone who's never smoked. After 10 years your lung cancer risk drops to nearly that of a non-smoker.

2. **Exercise daily**
   Thirty minutes of light activity is all that's necessary. Three 10-minute walks will do it.

3. **Eat five servings of fresh fruit/vegetables daily**
   These are full of antioxidants – the elite Army soldiers of protective nutrients. You want platoons of them deployed in your bloodstream at all times.

4. **Get screened**
   Elsewhere in this book we list the best health tests to get at different stages of life. Follow them.

5. **Get plenty of sleep**
   For most adults that means eight to nine hours every night. This is when your body's immune system reloads.

6. **Take a daily low-dose aspirin**
   Heart attack, stroke, even cancer… Just a single 75mg tablet per day appears to fight them all. But consult your doctor before you start, in case it conflicts with other medication.

7. **Know your blood pressure**

   It's not called the silent killer because our lives need more drama. Keep yours at around 120/80.

8. **Stay connected**

   Loneliness is another form of stress. Friends, family and furry pets supply vitamin F.

9. **Cut back on saturated fat**

   It's the raw material your body uses for producing bad (LDL) cholesterol.

10. **Get help for depression**

   As they say in *The Sopranos*, depression is rage turned inwards. It's self-destructive. In fact, when tagged onto diabetes or heart disease, it increases risk of early death by as much as 30 per cent.

11. **Manage stress**

   The doctors we surveyed claim that living with uncontrolled stress is more destructive to physical and mental health than being 15 kg overweight.

12. **Have a higher purpose**

   As one doctor advised, 'Strive to achieve something bigger than yourself.' Whether this happens via church, community or charity, when you give back, you also give to yourself.

YOU WON'T BE ALONE...

14,500 ▸ Estimated number of centenarians in the United Kingdom in 2012.

110,000 ▸ Projected number of centenarians in the UK in 2035, thanks both to better healthcare and people taking better care of themselves.

Raise a
fit child

A quarter of UK children are already overweight or obese when they start school at the age of four, and by the time they leave primary school at 11, the number rises to more than one in three. What has caused childhood obesity rates to rise so dramatically? Not McDonald's. Not Nintendo. Parents and grandparents are also to blame. We're the ones who teach, direct, inspire and shape. If you have a toddler who's become a waddler, or a teen who wears big jeans because they're practical rather than trendy, here's how to get 'em in shape.

Lead by example

Children learn by watching more than listening. So if your only exercise is couch surfing, don't expect them to grow up any differently. Prioritise working out and eating smart, and they will, too. It's that simple.

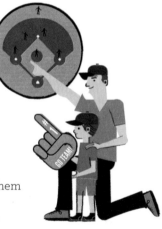

Emphasise activity over dieting

Restrictive fad diets are physically and mentally damaging to kids, depriving them of essential nutrients for development and setting them up for failure because they aren't long-term solutions. It's better to promote fitness and weight loss by encouraging them to move more. Notice we didn't use the word 'exercise'. To a youngster exercise is activity minus the fun. So sneak more movement into everyday life by walking or pedalling rather than driving, and planning active holidays rather than sedentary ones. Buy bikes instead of gaming systems. Be your family's activity coordinator.

Bring back home cooking

Kids are swallowing 31 per cent more calories, 56 per cent more fats and oils and 14 per cent more sugars and sweeteners than they were 40 years ago. A major reason is that the average British family spends about 30 per cent of its food budget at restaurants, where there's little control over what's ordered or how it's prepared. Save money and pounds by cooking more at home.

Improve snack quality

Forbidding kids to snack ultimately leads to sweet hoarding in the toy chest. Instead, make fresh fruit more available and cut it up. Buy microwave popcorn instead of crisps. And replace fizzy drinks with fresh fruit smoothies, milk and water (or any of the other healthy drinks listed on page 58). Kids are lazy; they'll grab what's available.

Never use food as a carrot

Buying him a Happy Meal or bar of chocolate every time he gets an A at school or scores a goal forever links fatty food with comfort in his subconscious. Instead, reward him verbally or with a healthy treat.

BRIBE 'EM! To give your gang more incentive to be active, create a reward system. Are the kids clamouring to go to Disneyland? Son wants a new skateboard? Make 'em earn it! Create a system that awards one point for each minute of activity, whether it's cycling or taking out the recycling. Or buy everyone a pedometer and tally total steps each day. Keep track of everyone's progress on a kitchen blackboard. By the time their goal is met, being more active will be a habit.

Make these health moves in
your 20s

What	When
Routine checks/exams	
Chlamydia test	Free on the NHS for under-25s
Blood pressure	Every 5 years
Cholesterol	Once *(if you have a family history of raised cholesterol or early cardiovascular disease)*
Blood glucose	Every 5 years *(every year if you have a family history of Type 1 diabetes or are overweight)*
Eyesight	Every 2 years
Teeth	At least every 2 years
Body mass index (BMI)	Annually
Testicular cancer	Monthly self-examination
Breast cancer	Monthly self-examination
Cervical smear	Every 3 years from the age of 25

Living well...

This is when the foundation for future youthfulness is laid. It's the decade for taking care of important long-term safeguards and cultivating good health habits. While it's not easy to prioritise health at such a seemingly invincible age, the steps taken now are no less important to eventual prosperity than starting a retirement savings plan.

Inoculations

Hepatitis B	Once per lifetime *(only for those at risk)*
Meningitis	Once per lifetime < age 25
Measles/mumps/rubella	Once *(if you weren't inoculated as a child)*
Tetanus-diphtheria	Check if you had the full five doses as a child, if not get it done now

General

Build strength.	Muscles are now at their developmental peak.
Line up a good GP surgery.	They'll be your lifetime advocates.
Do a family health history.	What killed Grandma could get you.

Never have a heart attack

Each year more than 200,000 people in the UK have heart attacks. Coronary heart disease is the commonest cause of premature death in the UK, but many first-time attacks are preventable. You already know about not smoking, avoiding saturated fat, reducing stress and losing weight, but here are some other important cornerstones of heart health you should be building upon.

Treat your heart like a muscle

That's because it is one. And by exercising it regularly and aerobically, you can increase its size; extreme athletes have been shown to increase theirs by 30 to 40 per cent. When you strengthen your heart, it's able to pump more blood with each stroke and doesn't need to beat as often overall. A lower pulse generally correlates with a healthier heart and a longer life. Swimmers, cross-country skiers, rowers and cyclists tend to have the largest hearts.

Take your medicine

Cholesterol-lowering statins, blood pressure medication and daily aspirin have all been proven safe and effective for reducing the risk of heart attack. Yet researchers found that most first-time heart-attack sufferers weren't taking advantage of them and, in most cases, may not even have been screened for cardiovascular disease. If you have a family history of heart trouble or other risk factors (overweight, smoker, stressed...), make sure you tell your doctor, who may want to check your blood pressure and cholesterol.

Add these items to your shopping list

Apples, almonds, avocados, bananas, barley, berries, broccoli, carrots, coffee (in moderation), kidney beans, kiwis, grape juice, lean beef, lentils, milk, mushrooms, porridge, olive oil, onions,

Living well...

papayas, pomegranate juice, red wine, spinach, sweet potatoes, tea (green, white, black, oolong), tomatoes, turkey, walnuts, watermelon, wild salmon and (yes!) dark chocolate. Because of the special nutrients (chiefly antioxidants and fibre) they contain, all these foods are extremely heart healthy. By the way, science now recommends getting nutrients naturally via food rather than in pill form. Our bodies don't seem to utilise most nutrients the same way when swallowed as supplements.

Live a life of 'we,' not 'me'

According to research, the more frequently a person uses 'self-referencing' words, such as I, me, and my, the greater their risk of having a heart attack. Seems odd, but it turns out that emotional connection – not separateness – is good for the heart in more ways than one. Research shows that a strong support network of friends and family, along with a charitable and optimistic mindset, lowers stress, boosts immunity and even hastens recovery if you do get sick.

THE TICKER

▶▶ **100,000** = number of times your heart beats in one day

▶▶ **35 million** = number of times your heart beats in one year

▶▶ **2.5 billion** = number of times your heart beats in a lifetime

▶▶ **10 pints** = amount of blood in the human body

▶▶ **20 seconds** = time it takes for all that blood to circulate through the body

▶▶ **12,000 miles** = distance that blood travels in one day

▶▶ **1 million** = number of barrels of blood pumped in one lifetime

▶▶ **3** = number of supertankers those barrels would fill

Avoid food-borne illness

When you think of dangerous foods, deep-fried Mars bars and megaburgers typically come to mind but they're not the only threat. The FSA estimated that in in 2007 around a million people in the UK suffered a food-borne illness (food poisoning), leading to 20,000 receiving hospital treatment and 500 deaths. Here are some of the non-meat culprits for many incidences of food-borne illness reported each year, along with how to avoid being victimised by each.

Berries
Nooks and crannies provide hideouts for bad guys. Depending on the fruit's fragility, soak, spray or scrub with fresh water. Avoid ordering in restaurants where the likelihood of a good cleaning is low.

Bean sprouts
Since being identified in 2011 as the probable source of a deadly E. coli outbreak that killed 22 people and made more than 2,000 ill across Europe, sprouts have been shown to be challenging to distribute safely and clean. Best avoided.

Tomatoes
Don't buy ones with splits or cracks (windows for salmonella) or eat them fresh at restaurants (many outbreaks occur there). Otherwise, wash well in water.

Ice cream
Soft-serve is particularly hazardous because bacterium often thrives in the dispensing machines. If you're making your own ice cream, try to use recipes that skip the raw egg.

Cheese
As with ice cream, it's mostly the soft varieties that trouble stomachs. Brie, Camembert, feta and anything homemade should be approached with caution.

Living well...

Potatoes

Grandma was right: beware the potato salad. Forty per cent of outbreaks involving spuds originate in restaurants and grocery delis because of improper storage.

Oysters

These bivalves can contain the same family of bacterium as cholera. Slurp some soup as an appetiser instead.

Tuna

Approximately 65 per cent of illnesses from this fish can be traced back to restaurants. So if you're craving tuna salad or a nice fillet, make it yourself and cook the tuna thoroughly.

Eggs

Never eat raw or runny ones, and avoid indulging in eggs (or egg dishes) at breakfast buffets or catered events, where warming temperatures may be inadequate.

Leafy greens

How can something so nutritious be atop a most-dangerous foods list? The simple reason is, greens often aren't washed properly, if at all. The FDA says to be particularly wary of restaurant salads and to always clean prepackaged supermarket greens even if the label says 'prewashed'.

WHAT NOT TO DO IF YOU'RE HIT... Something you ate turning your stomach? Skip the anti-diarrhoea pills. You want that bug, whatever it is, out of you pronto. By resorting to Imodium or other similar medicines, you could slow its passage and worsen your condition. Most cases of food poisoning last less than 48 hours, during which time you should rest and stay hydrated. Anything beyond that needs a doctor's expertise.

Boost your immunity

If your mother was anything like ours, then staying healthy was a simple matter of 'Don't get your feet wet!' and 'Do up your coat!' Although science disproved those two warnings long ago – along with 'Some day your face will freeze like that!' – some of mum's favourite threats about avoiding impending death did turn out to be correct. To bolster your body's defence against germs and illness, try listening to her for once.

'Don't be such a misery!'
'Happier people are less likely to develop colds when exposed to cold viruses,' says Sheldon Cohen, PhD, a professor of psychology at Carnegie Mellon University. Even the simple act of smiling fights infection.

'Go and play outside!'
Regular exercise increases the number of disease-fighting cells patrolling the bloodstream. And if you exercise outdoors for 10 or 15 minutes before applying sunscreen, you'll also get an immunity-boosting dose of vitamin D (the sunshine vitamin), which is low in 50 per cent of adults.

'Eat your vegetables!'
The brightest and deepest coloured ones have the most antioxidants. But if stuff like spinach still makes you grimace, 'hide' a nice assortment of them – plus health-ensuring onions, garlic and tomatoes – in a pot of homemade vegetarian chilli. Top each bowl with a dollop of probiotic-rich Greek yogurt. It's the new chicken soup.

'Be nice to your brother!'

Charitable acts raise levels of immunoglobulin A, an antibody in saliva that fights infection. In fact, just observing or considering generosity does it. When university students watched a documentary of Mother Teresa ministering to the sick, they enjoyed the same effect.

'Go wash your hands!'

Despite how clichéd it sounds, this is the single best thing you can do to stay healthy. Either use alcohol-based gels, or scrub for 20 seconds with soap and water. And then keep your fingers out of your mouth!

'It'll only hurt for a little while!'

Thanks to vaccination, we no longer see smallpox in the UK, and polio and whooping cough are heading towards eradication. See the vaccination checklist at www.nhs.uk to find out which ones you and your family should ideally have.

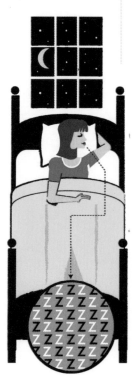

'Go to bed, now!'

Not getting the recommended seven and a half to nine hours of sleep per night raises your risk of colds, flu, obesity, diabetes, heart disease and even cancer. As an example of just how important rest is to health, a University of Chicago study found that men with no risk factors for diabetes were in a pre-diabetic state after just one week of poor sleep. (See 'Sleep Well Tonight (and Every Night)', page 12.)

SURPRISING THINGS YOU CAN CATCH It's not just the sniffles and conjunctivities that are contagious. Apparently, so is:

▸▸ **Obesity** Adenovirus-36 is more likely to be found in the obese than the thin. And when lab animals are exposed to this virus, they begin gaining weight. Although more research is needed, the theory is that some viruses might infect cells and cause them to store fat.

▸▸ **Heart attack** Myocarditis is an inflammation of the heart muscle that can be triggered by a range of viral infections (cold, mononucleosis, measles and HIV as well as bacterial infections.) If you have a stubborn illness, see a doctor before it works its way into your heart.

▸▸ **Divorce** According to research at the University of California, San Diego, the breakup of friends increases your chance of divorce by 147 per cent. Psychologists call it 'divorce clustering' and speculate that it encourages an if-they-can-so-can-I attitude.

▸▸ **Emotions** Other people's moods can infect yours. A study even quantified it: one sad friend doubles your chance of also becoming sad. And for each happy friend you have, your chance of personal happiness rises by 11 per cent.

Lower your stress by
75 per cent

You've heard the scary statistics – how millions fall victim to heart disease, stroke and cancer every year. In fact, you're probably reading this book in the hopes of finding the key to minimising your risk. Well, here it is: lower your stress. Stress is a major underlying cause of disease and deterioration, both physical and mental. Yet in our misguided minds we've come to accept it as a normal part of modern life. While it's true that some stress is necessary for success (it pushes us), we're way over the healthy limit. Here are the simplest and best ways we've found to manage it.

Learn to say no
Much of stress is self-inflicted. It comes from being too nice and trying to do too much. To instantly cure yourself of this, repeat these five words politely after us: 'Sorry, I'm too busy now.'

Cry in the shower
We knew a woman who would take a shower in difficult times and cry her heart out. By the time she stepped out, she was cleansed – literally and emotionally – and felt better able to face the day and other people. Despite how imbalanced this seems, having an emotional outlet rebalanced her.

Or try a smile
You can get angry at the unfairness of it all, or you can laugh it off, because you just can't control what others say or do, and getting angry achieves nothing. This takes practice, but in time you really can train yourself to react to the craziness of life with health-preserving zen.

Create pockets of peace

Beyond caffeine and nicotine, there's an army of everyday stimulants most people are largely unaware of. Traffic noise, background music, television, the internet, machinery, crowds, harsh lighting... It's all stress inducing. Withstand the assault by creating (and savouring) pockets of peace in daily life. Roll up the car windows and turn off the radio. Remove televisions and computers from the bedroom. Eat more quiet dinners at home rather than at noisy restaurants. Deem one day per week information-free and don't use the internet. Learn to cherish these oases of calm.

Drop your shoulders

Buy a pack of Post-it notes in some nice bright colour. Write three words ('Drop Your Shoulders') on a dozen or so and stick them throughout your life – on your car's dashboard, inside a kitchen cabinet, on the computer monitor... Most of us live with our shoulders up around our ears, which causes headaches and neck pain. These little reminders will end that bad habit and have an amazing calming effect. The same trick works if you channel your angst in other physical habits, be it slouching, biting your nails or playing with your hair.

Do savasana anytime

Yoga classes traditionally end with a period of relaxation called savasana. You lie on your back, close your eyes, clear your mind and dip into the first stages of restorative sleep. Although it only lasts a few minutes, it feels delicious. But it doesn't have to be done in the context of yoga. Just close the office door or lie down on your living-room rug any time you feel like it, reminding yourself that you're not a human *doing*, you're a human *being*.

NERVES OF SEAL One of the first things US Navy SEALs, military pilots and bomb techs master is how to remain calm under pressure. No surprise there. But what is surprising is the remarkably simple way they learn this. Lieutenant Colonel David Grossman, who trains them all, begins with a lesson in breathing. The more excited or stressed you are, he explains, the quicker and shallower your respiration and the higher your blood pressure and heart rate. Most people live in this state of alert 24/7, which compromises physical and mental performance, in addition to health.

To begin changing how you breathe, do this: put your hand on your belly and breathe normally. You'll probably notice that very little is happening down there. Now try letting your belly expand like a balloon as you inhale slowly through your nose, then let it deflate as you exhale. That's how you should be breathing all the time. The additional oxygen will nourish every cell in your body and ease your stress.

Flatten your stomach

No health book would be complete without this promise. If you believe the magazines and adverts, this is the key to success and (of course) incredible sex. But let's be realistic. Given the cruel fact that the only time most of us will ever sport a six-pack is when we're carrying one home from the off-licence, a different strategy is in order. Forget about crunches. Resist the urge to order the latest miracle machine by calling the freephone number on your screen. Instead, start whittling away your middle this way.

Assess the job
Wrap a tape measure snugly around your waist, just above the hipbones. According to the NHS, anything over 80cm for women and 94cm for men means you have a higher risk of health problems and deserves your immediate attention.

Get the right motivation
From a health perspective belly fat is the worst kind to be saddled with. Because it's visceral (meaning it surrounds internal organs), it can increase your risk for heart disease, stroke, diabetes and cancer. So flattening your tummy isn't solely an exercise in vanity; it's about health and living longer. And you don't have to get cover-model abs to enjoy the benefits. (There, pressure's off.)

Remember, 'First to arrive, last to leave'
Fat is the ultimate bad guest. The first place it gets deposited, which is usually around the waist, is the last place it exits. So despite what the magazine covers say, you're not going to lose your gut in seven days. Try taking the long view instead: more like seven *months*.

Forget about spot reduction

It's impossible to turn fat into muscle. You could do a million sit-ups, but all that will do is make the ab muscles lying beneath your belly fat stronger. You lose belly fat by losing weight. And the best exercises for that are ones that burn the most calories, namely, aerobic activities that work the entire body.

Pull everybody's eyes up

An ornate belt or buckle, or bangles when your arms are by your sides, draws attention to your middle. Instead, wear a nice necklace, earrings or bright shirt to keep the focus up.

Wear something naughty underneath

Slimming undergarments have come a long way since girdles and corsets. In fact, body-shaping compression wear is one of the fastest-growing clothing categories for women *and* men. Go ahead, wear those control pants – we won't tell anyone.

DRESS 10 POUNDS THINNER Since it takes time to lose a tummy, here are some additional dress-slimmer tips from fashion expert Stacy London:

▸▸ Instead of letting shirts hang down to your thighs, keep them at hip height. 'It helps you look taller and leaner by maintaining a long leg line,' she explains.

▸▸ As long as the belt doesn't have a flashy buckle that calls immediate attention to your middle, it's okay to wear one. Contrary to popular belief, London says that having a belt subtly cut across your middle helps shorten the torso and creates a longer, slimming leg line.

▸▸ In colder weather wear a sweater and keep your coat open. With a longer-style coat, this will create a vertical line that makes you look taller and thinner.

Save your marriage,
save your health

Among all the things prescribed to better our health – exercise, weight loss, low-fat eating, check-ups – rarely, if ever, are we advised to work on our marriages. Yet various studies have shown that an unhappy marriage increases your chance of getting sick by as much as 35 per cent and shortens your life by up to four years. Researchers have even found that happily married men and women have more white blood cells and natural killer cells in their bodies, which boosts immunity. Hmmm. Maybe it's time to take some new vows.

Exercise less

This is the only time you'll ever hear us advocate this, but marriage researcher John Gottman, PhD, makes sense when he says, 'If fitness buffs spent just 10 per cent of their weekly workout time – say, 20 minutes a day – working on their marriage instead of their bodies, they would get three times the health benefits.' Think of it as *marital* fitness.

Kiss hello, kiss goodbye

Parting with a kiss in the morning and greeting each other with a kiss in the evening is one of the simplest ways for couples to stay connected on a daily basis. Think you're too old for that routine to make sparks fly? Rub your stocking feet on the carpet just prior to puckering up and a tiny bit of static electricity will leap from lip to lip. Yeah, you still got it.

Stop keeping score

With all due respect to Father O'Malley, marriage is not a 50/50 proposition. If you're keeping tabs on whether your spouse polished the wheel rims after you waxed the car, then, says Dr Gottman, 'you're probably not in love anymore.'

Don't withdraw in a fight

Giving your spouse the silent treatment after a disagreement can be just as toxic to a relationship as yelling or calling each other names in a knock-down, drag-out battle royale, researchers have found. 'Successful couples know how to exit an argument,' says Dr. Gottman. Strategies include making a caring remark, offering signs of appreciation for your spouse or simply agreeing this is 'our' problem.

Teach your dog a new trick

Humour and distraction are also great ways to defuse an argument. Here's a novel idea that supplies both: think of the phrases that you and your spouse typically use during a fight. Then start repeating these whenever you play ball with your dog. In time ol' Roscoe (that's the dog, not your spouse) will recognise these 'commands', grab the ball and hopefully defuse the disagreement. Now, don't scoff; this is a *lot* cheaper than therapy.

> # 100 beats per minute
> ➤ The heart rate at which arguing couples begin having trouble processing what their partner is saying.

Pour more of these
healthy drinks

Cola, bad. Fruit squash, bad. Sweetened teas, bad. Beer, *very* bad. Talk to someone who's serious about health and they'll tell you that many popular drinks are bad for you and that you should live mostly on iced water and hot tea. Don't take them seriously, either. There are lots of drinks that are perfectly fine for you, such as...

Sparkling fruit juice

One hundred per cent juices, such as pomegranate, blueberry, grape, apple, orange and blackcurrant are full of disease-fighting nutrients. But they're also high in calories from natural sugars and can prompt weight gain if enjoyed often. The perfect compromise? Mix 20–25ml of juice with 250ml of sparkling water. It tastes like soda but is much more refreshing and healthy.

Low-sodium vegetable juice cocktail

If you have the time to juice your own vegetables, then more power to you. If not, low-sodium V8 is a good alternative, especially if you have a family history of heart disease. Marie Almon, MS, RD, a US nutrition director, recommends small cartons of vegetable juice blends. Low-sodium V8 is a good alternative, especially if you have a family history of heart disease. One 50-calorie serving contains heart-healthy fibre, lycopene, potassium and vitamins A and C, while supplying less sugar than the same amount of orange juice and a not-bad 140mg of sodium.

Infused water

You'll find this offered at luxury spas, but there's no reason why you can't indulge at home. Simply fill a small jug with water and add prewashed fruit (lemon, berries), herbs (mint, lemongrass), or something creative (cucumber, ginger). Let it steep in the fridge overnight. Imagine you're at Champneys.

POUR LESS

Energy drinks Brands such as Red Bull, Monster and Relentless provide energy in unhealthy amounts from unhealthy sources. Energy drinks contain high levels of caffeine and sugar, while many other ingredients that are claimed to give you a lift are unregulated. But caffeine is the real culprit. An average 250ml can contains 80mg of caffeine, the same amount as three cans of cola. In high doses it has been associated with anxiety, poor concentration, seizures, stomach upset, insomnia and palpitations, and could even raise the risk of heart disease and stroke. Energy drinks are not recommended for children or pregnant women and are not great for the rest of us either.

Fancy coffees A Grande drink at Starbucks is a meal in a cup. It's not surprising that the UK's collective rise in weight has coincided with the growth of its coffee cups.

▶▶ **Starbucks White Chocolate Mocha Frappuccino** (c.470ml with whole milk and whipped cream) = calorie equivalent (440) of a McDonald's Double Cheeseburger.

Fruit smoothie

When ordered out, this is often a health-food imposter. A small McDonald's Wild Berry Smoothie, for example, contains about the same amount of sugar (44g) as a can of cola. But if you make one at home with fresh, low-fat ingredients and no added sugar, it can be a nutritious and satisfying meal replacement. Combine ice, low-fat yogurt, bananas, strawberries, mangoes or whatever else fits your taste and imagination. Kids love to make them, too.

Soup
Most people don't think of soup as a drink, but it *is,* and it's extremely healthy when homemade. Keep a stock of low-fat, low-sodium vegetable or chicken stockcubes. For a warming meal or snack, make a broth and add frozen vegetables and whole-wheat pasta or brown rice.

Chocolate milk
Your childhood favourite can still be your adult favourite. Personal trainers actually recommend low-fat chocolate milk as a recovery drink because of the protein and other nutrients it supplies. It's also rich in calcium and vitamin D, which fights osteoporosis, and if you mix your own using unsweetened cocoa powder, there's even evidence it aids the cardiovascular system by reducing inflammation. Plus, you always looked good with a moustache.

Managing
the system

Stress is a major underlying cause of disease and death, which is why it's so ironic (and sad) that our healthcare system is dispensing so much of it. If you're often frustrated, confused or overwhelmed by medical and dietary options, this section will show you how to gain more control and make smarter decisions. Whether you're trying to find the best doctors or vitamins, a top-notch surgeon or workout, consider this your GPS for getting where you want to go with minimal hassle.

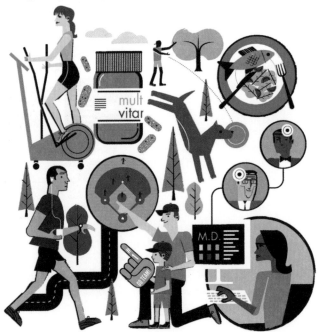

Find a
top-notch doctor

The partner who has the most potential to influence your life is not the one sleeping beside you every night. Rather, it's one most people choose with far less care than the decision deserves. We're talking about your family doctor – the general practitioner who is the first line in your health defence and, thus, your *real* life partner. Here's how to find one you love.

See what's possible

Most GPs operate a catchment area, so begin by getting a list of doctors from your local library or consulting the telephone directory. Alternatively, go online and enter your postcode in the NSH Choices Find Services system (nhs.uk/ServiceDirectories/), which also allows patients to rate doctors. Then you'll need to ring up or check the practice's website and find out if you live in the area it covers and if they're taking on new patients.

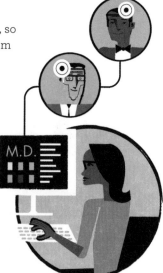

Ask around

Friends, family, neighbours, colleagues, other doctors, nurses, even local blogs and forums, are all great sources for referrals. There are also websites that allow patients to review GPs or surgeries, including Iwantgreatcare.org and Patientopinion.org.uk.

Check the record

See if the doctors you're considering are licensed to practise and whether they've had any disciplinary action taken against them by taking a look at the General Medical Council's list of registered medical practitioners (gmc-uk.org/register, or call the GMC on 0161 923 6602). The list also specifies if a doctor has a specialty. Then search the names of doctors you're considering on the internet. Although you can't trust everything there, it may turn up additional insights. If a named GP and continuity of care are important to you, it might be worth opting for a doctor who is a member of the Family Doctor Association. Their website (family-doctor.org.uk) has a search facility.

'Never go to a doctor whose office plants have died.'

– Erma Bombeck

Go undercover

Call the surgery of each doctor on your shortlist and ask some basic questions, such as if they're open in the evening and at weekends or whether any of the doctors have special interests (useful information if you have a particular condition). More important than the answers is how long it takes to get a real person on the line and how pleasant and efficient they seem. Then visit the surgery to see what kind of vibe you get. How long does it take before someone greets you? Does the staff look happy and in control? What's the mood in the waiting room?

Look for a connection

When you get to see your new GP, note whether he or she runs behind schedule. Doctors are extremely busy, but does she look you in the eyes and listen?

Be persistent

If the doctor you want is not taking new patients, that's a good sign. It might be worth trying again at a later date, or asking if there is a waiting list you can join.

Spend less time in hospital

Nobody – well hardly anybody – wants to spend any more time than necessary in hospital. However nice the nursing staff and however much you enjoy watching *Holby City*, the reality is that the longer you stay, the more chances there are for problems to occur. To lower the risk of being prescribed the wrong drugs, left in a corridor or infected with a superbug, follow these simple rules.

Stay away in August

During their junior years, most doctors change jobs at intervals of between six months and two years. The peak changeover period, when they all seem to switch jobs at once, is in August. This is the month when most newly qualified doctors – those who were mere medical students a few months before and those moving up to higher grades or to a different specialty – take on their new roles. Apparently, it's also the month in which the highest number of medical errors usually occur. Mistakes in writing out prescriptions are especially common at this time. Many hospitals have systems in place to help those who have only just taken up their posts, but if you can wait until September for that much-needed hip replacement, you might be better off.

Avoid weekends

Unless it's really an emergency – if you're just having tests or elective surgery – try to avoid being admitted to hospital at the weekend or on a public holiday. A survey by the Dr Foster Unit at Imperial College, London, showed that mortality rates in hospitals generally rise steadily from their lowest level on Tuesdays to their highest point on Sundays, before dropping back sharply on Mondays. 'We found that death rates for elective and emergency admissions increased by 7 per cent over the weekend,' said Professor Sir Brian Jarman, who led the research. He strongly suspects that the lower staffing levels at weekends and at holiday times are the underlying cause of these variations.

Check for clean hands

Hand-washing before and after contact with a patient is the main recommended method for reducing the spread of infections in hospitals. Yet a study carried out at the University of Hertfordshire found that 88 per cent of hospital staff frequently didn't bother. A quarter of them didn't even clean their hands properly after they had been handling human waste. No wonder the UK has high rates of hospital-borne infections, such as the MRSA 'superbug'. Not washing your hands 'is the clinical equivalent of drink driving. It maims and kills,' according to Sir John Oldham, a government adviser on primary healthcare. So don't feel nervous or embarrassed about asking nurses, doctors and other hospital staff to wash their hands before they touch you – it could save your life.

Learn to avoid blood clots

Around one in ten of all hospital deaths in Britain are thought to be caused by pulmonary embolism – blood clots on the lungs. Clots often form in the lower legs when a patient has to lie still in bed for long periods. This is known as deep vein thrombosis or DVT – the same problem that can arise when flying long distances in the cramped conditions of economy class. These clots can break away and travel in the bloodstream to the lungs, causing a fatal blockage. People over 40, and those having surgery on the abdomen, hips or legs, are especially at risk. Lifeblood, the thrombosis charity, offers information about DVT and advises anyone who is about to go into hospital to speak to their medical team about the risk of blood clots and measures they can take to avoid them.

Best 20 minute workout:
Interval training

To get the most benefit from limited exercise time, do interval training, says Arthur Agastson, the heart doctor who founded the South Beach Diet. This involves systematically raising and lowering your heart rate over the course of a workout. Doing so has many benefits: Interval training strengthens the cardiovascular system, burns additional calories and fat, combats boredom, boosts fitness and lowers insulin levels/resistance. Plus, the concept can be applied to just about any activity, from walking or biking to using indoor machines like stationary bikes. Here's a simple schedule you can follow (once you're cleared by your doctor). There's no need for a heart-rate monitor, just base your pace on 'perceived exertion' or how you feel.

1. *Warm up for 3 minutes at a comfortable pace.*

2. *Do six 30-second intervals, alternating 15 seconds at a faster pace with 15 seconds at normal pace.*

3. *Do eight 60-second intervals, alternating 30 seconds at a faster pace with 30 seconds at normal pace.*

4. *Do six 30-second intervals, alternating 15 seconds at a faster pace with 15 seconds at normal pace.*

5. *Cool down for 3 minutes at a comfortable pace.*

6. *Do this workout every other day, adjusting the number and length of the intervals as your fitness improves.*

PERSONAL N●TES

{ How can I get **more movement** into my day? }

Make sense
of media health reports

One day eggs are bad for you; the next day they're beneficial. One day vitamin E supplements are great for the heart; the next day they're not. On one visit your doctor tells you to boost good cholesterol, but on another he's not even sure it's 'good' anymore. The list goes on. It seems that practically every week there's another news report about a study contradicting some aspect of healthy living previously considered gospel. If you're increasingly frustrated and confused by this, a little perspective can go a long way.

Don't immediately swallow it

Despite being performed by MDs and PhDs, health studies are often initially interpreted by reporters with far less expertise. Plus, the unfortunate inclination of today's media is to sensationalise things, especially on websites, where boosting page views and beating the competition are paramount. So don't practice knee-jerk medicine by starting (or stopping) anything based on a first report.

Study the study

ScienceDaily.com provides accurate and balanced study summaries, plus links to the source of the story. Bookmark it. To have merit, a study must meet certain criteria: it should be conducted by a reputable person or organisation (the National Institute for Health and Clinical Excellence or Marie Stopes International, for instance). It should be (or is about to be) published in a respected, peer-reviewed journal (e.g. *The Lancet*). It should use a fairly large sample (thousands rather than dozens) of humans (not lab animals). And it should be independent (free of influence from sponsors with vested interests). If any of these conditions are not met, be suspect.

Wait for reaction

Single studies rarely change medicine. In the weeks following the initial report, doctors and other experts will interpret the findings and put them in context with other research. Unfortunately, this perspective is not usually reported at the same fever pitch, if at all. So wait a week or two and then Google 'reaction/implications to XXX study' to determine what to do.

Accept that science is fluid

As technology advances, it allows us to examine things in new ways. Pluto, for example, is no longer a planet, and we now know that bacteria rather than stress cause ulcers. So don't view shifting science as evidence of disarray and allow it to demoralise you. Instead, welcome it as refinement and, with the help of your doctor, apply it.

SO IS IT GOOD OR BAD?

▸▸ **Butter:** High in cholesterol and saturated fat. Minimise.

▸▸ **Margarine:** Trans fat-free spreads or oils such as olive, rapeseed or sunflower are a better choice than butter.

▸▸ **Eggs:** No more than four yolks per week, if you're cholesterol sensitive.

▸▸ **Coffee:** One or two cups per day of regular are fine, but decaf is best.

▸▸ **Meat:** Okay if it's lean and skin removed from chicken.

Buy the best
vitamins

How big is the health supplements industry? Let's put it this way: British consumers spend more than £170 million every year on vitamins and supplements. Yet regulation in this market is complex, with some products classified as medicines being regulated very carefully and others classed as supplements facing no safety or quality checks at all. Recent studies have raised doubts about the effectiveness of such bestsellers as multivitamins, antioxidants and even vitamin C. To be sure you're taking quality products that will improve rather than hurt your health, here's what to do.

Think big picture

Vitamins and supplements may not be medicine, but they're still pills that introduce chemicals into your body. And that means they can interact with one another and prescription medications. For instance, if you're taking calcium to prevent osteoporosis, are you aware it could reduce the effectiveness of some antibiotics? Likewise, fish oil can interfere with some blood-pressure drugs. So everything you're taking must be viewed in concert. The American National Institutes of Health's website medlineplus.gov lists the efficacy, safety concerns, and side effects of 100 popular herbs and supplements. Use this information and the advice of your doctor to decide what (if anything) you should take.

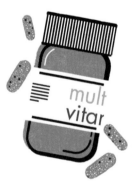

Buying safely

Any vitamin or herbal product making a medical claim has to be licensed as a medicine and undergo rigorous quality, safety and efficacy tests (look out for a PL number on the label). For herbal medicines, find one that is part of the Traditional Herbal Registration Scheme and you can be assured that the product has gone through safety and quality checks (look out for the THR logo or THR number on products). Be wary of anything classified as a supplement as there is no regulation of these by an external body. To ensure you choose safely, buy from a pharmacist who will have bought from a reputable source and can advise on correct dosage.

VITAMIN BS

One-Third »The amount of supplements analysed by consumer groups that contained doses much lower or higher than stated on their labels.

Do the vinegar test

We have a friend who once had a CT scan that showed a blotch in her lower intestine. She was relieved but surprised to learn it was an undigested multivitamin. To be sure your supplements are dissolving inside you as they're supposed to, drop one of each in a glass of vinegar. If they're still there 30 minutes later, they're just commuting through your small intestine, where most nutrients are absorbed, and you should try another brand.

Get what you need from food

When it comes to supplements, there may very well be no magic pill. Scientists are finding that when micronutrients like antioxidants are isolated and taken on their own, they don't have the same health benefits as when they're consumed naturally in food. So the smartest plan of all may be what you've known all along: eat as varied a diet as possible of whole foods, fresh fruit and vegetables.

Outsmart
a restaurant menu

Seventy-one per cent of adults say they're trying to eat more healthily at restaurants, according to a recent poll. But good intention and resisting temptation are two entirely different things. For proof, look around the next time you're at one of those Chinese buffets and see how many people are loading up on steamed tofu. If you travel a lot for business or eat out frequently with family and friends, here's how to stick to your guns and finally tighten that tummy.

Take home half of what you order

If you're at a restaurant that's renowned for its large portions, don't feel obliged to finish it all. Doggy bags are part and parcel of eating out in the US, but many British diners struggle with the idea of asking to take their leftovers home. Be brave and ask the waiter to put half your meal in a takeaway container *before* she brings it to the table. This will ensure you don't overeat – and you'll end up with a ready-made lunch for the next day.

Create your own Special of the Day

A menu is really just an organised inventory of what's in the kitchen. You're free to have those ingredients prepared or paired any way you like. So order the fish grilled with lemon rather than fried in butter, swap the creamy coleslaw for a side salad and ask for a baked potato rather than French fries – in other words, *you* be the chef.

Use these tricks at the trough

All-you-can-eat restaurants are generally the least healthy dining-out option. But if you find yourself at one, try to sit facing away from the buffet. Be sure to browse the food first; otherwise, you'll just keep piling food on your plate as you encounter items you like. Also choose the smallest serving plate available. And when it's finally time to eat, put a napkin on your lap (for some reason, it makes you less likely to keep getting up for more). Researchers have found that doing all these things significantly reduces the amount of food you eat.

Make a meal of starters

These are usually smaller portions, and there are a lot to choose from on most menus. So make believe you're at a Spanish tapas restaurant and order two or three as your main meal.

Leave less room for treacle tart

If dessert is your downfall, order a bowl of healthy soup (tomato, vegetable) or a slice of bread with two tablespoons of dipping olive oil as your starter. Either option will fill you up so you'll eat less later. In fact, olive oil prompts the release of a stomach hormone called cholecystokinin, which suppresses appetite.

NEVER ORDER THIS

▸▸ **Chicken Korma:** With naan, it's around 1,300 calories.

▸▸ **Rib of Beef:** A typical cut has as many calories and as much fat as a Big Mac.

▸▸ **Caesar Salad:** Can be up to 80 per cent fat because of all the oil and cheese it's pre-tossed with.

▸▸ **Nachos:** Melted cheese on top of fatty beef on top of fried chips. A few chopped tomatoes and onions can't rescue that.

▸▸ **Pizza with the works:** Sausage, pepperoni and salami are among the fattiest meats on the planet.

Wait less
in waiting rooms

One of the underlying reasons many people don't take better care of themselves is because the process of seeing a doctor can be interminable. You have to jockey for an appointment weeks in advance, take time off from work, then sit (and sit) in a room surrounded by patients (and old magazines) you hope aren't contagious. Here are the best ways we've found to spend far less time waiting in waiting rooms.

Book a telephone appointment
Ask the receptionist if your doctor does telephone consultations. If so he'll be able to answer your questions, sign you off work, review test results and even discuss your symptoms over the phone, without you needing to go anywhere.

Book these slots
If a face-to-face consultation is necessary, try to reserve the first or second appointment of the day to minimise the risk of being delayed. The first slot after lunch is also good (if the doctor breaks for one). Bonus: you may even get better care because the staff are fresher.

Call ahead
If you have an appointment later in the day, call the surgery an hour before leaving to see if the doctor is on schedule. If not, delay your arrival accordingly. For an Accident & Emergency visit that doesn't involve a life-threatening situation, go around 9.00 A.M., when it's usually calmer.

Visit the chemist

For minor infections, injuries and advice on how to stop smoking, visit one of the NHS walk-in centres that have opened recently in local hospitals, GP surgeries and even some branches of Boots. They're usually staffed by a nurse, have convenient hours and are open 365 days a year. But what's most attractive is that no appointment is necessary. Private walk-in clinics, staffed by doctors and usually found in larger towns, have also gained in popularity in the past few years and you can now even book a Skype GP consultation through Lloyds Pharmacy private online doctor service.

DON'T MIND WAITING Instead of stressing out about waiting, treat it as an opportunity to relax – some precious downtime in your demanding day. Start the novel you've been anxious to read, watch a film on your laptop, listen to a lecture on your mobile or iPod (earplugs please!), or just close your eyes and take a nap. It isn't a disruption; it's a gift.

Make these health moves in
your **30s**

What	When
Routine checks/exams	
Blood pressure	Every 5 years
Cholesterol	Once *(if you have a family history of raised cholesterol or early cardiovascular disease)*
Blood glucose	Every 5 years *(every year if you have a family history of Type 1 diabetes or are overweight)*
Eyesight	Every 2 years
Teeth	At least every 2 years *(seek guidance from your dentist)*
Body mass index (BMI)	Every 6 months
Testicular cancer	Monthly self-examination
Breast cancer	Monthly self-examination
Cervical smear test	Every 3 years

Managing the system

his go-go decade of career- and family-building is when many root causes of disease gain a foothold. These include chronic stress, inadequate sleep, poor nutrition and weight gain. While it's not easy to find time for yourself amid everything else, the less you let slip away now the less you'll have to make up later.

Inoculations

Various	If missed in prior decade (see page 42)

General

Find a life partner.	Married people live longer.
Manage stress.	Nothing is more debilitating long term.
Prioritise sleep.	Adults need 8 to 9 hours nightly... *really*.
Eat smart to control weight.	Metabolism is on the decline.
Enjoy your endurance.	It peaks during this decade.

Negotiate
Accident & Emergency

Two hours and 26 minutes. That's the average time you can expect to spend hanging around in a hospital casualty department (though much longer waits are not unknown). To put this in perspective, that's just enough time to fly from London to Rome or almost as long as Britney Spears and Jason Alexander were married. Here's how to get in and out of A&E with the care you need much more efficiently.

Head out of central London
A & E patients at hospitals in the heart of the capital waited the longest of anywhere according to 2010/2011 figures – an average of 6 hours, 51 minutes.

Do your homework
Not all hospitals have Accident and Emergency departments, so find out which ones in your area do, before an emergency happens. Do this by 1) putting your postcode into the Services Search facility on the NHS Choices website (nhs.uk/servicedirectories) which also has patient reviews on individual hospitals' pages, or 2) calling NHS Direct on 0845 46 47 in England and Wales and NHS 24 on 08454 24 24 24 in Scotland.

Make sure you're in the right place
The reason wait times are so long is because A&Es are overwhelmed (often, the delay is finding beds in a hospital for admitted patients). If there's a life-threatening situation (loss of consciousness, signs of heart attack or stroke, severe pain, heavy bleeding) don't hesitate in getting to one. But if it's a minor burn, bite, break, illness or irritation, save time by visiting a minor injuries unit, usually based in a local hospital. Find your nearest

one by using the services search facility on the NHS Choices website (nhs.uk). These units offer a middle ground between doctors' surgeries and emergency departments. You can also call 111, the new free NHS number if you need medical help fast but it's not a life-or-death emergency. If in doubt about what to do in a non–life threatening situation, contact your doctor.

Call an ambulance

If it's a serious situation, the ambulance crew will not only start treatment but also call ahead so the hospital is prepared for your arrival. That saves critical time compared to just showing up.

Practise full disclosure

No matter how embarrassing or intimate the accident or affliction, telling the medical staff everything will get you faster, more focused care. This extends to health history, current medications and even supplements you're taking. Consider wearing a medical ID bracelet or necklace in case you're unconscious. New models contain downloadable flash drives.

Look on the bright side

The longer you're kept waiting, the less serious your condition probably is. It's the grave situations that get treated first. Nonetheless, don't be shy about periodically checking with the nurses as to when you'll be seen, but make sure to do it politely.

MOST COMMON A&E ERROR? Medication mistakes. To protect yourself amid all the commotion, get the nurse or doctor to do a double check by asking what the medication is, who it's for and why you're getting it. Asking these three simple questions will prevent most errors.

Take your
medicine

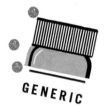

GENERIC

When your doctor prescribes a drug, that's just the beginning. Actually getting the medicine, not to mention taking it as directed, for the full course, are all crucial parts of the process that many of us seem to overlook as soon as we start to feel a bit better. But to get the most from your medicine, you have to take it – all of it.

Check your medicine

Before you leave the chemist's counter, check the medicine you've been given and, if you have any doubts about it being correct, ask: 'Is this what my doctor prescribed?' One study involving 23 doctors in three general practices found that 7.46 per cent of prescriptions contained an error. Mistakes were most common in those that were handwritten rather than computer-generated.

Read the ingredients lists

If your child has the sniffles, you may be tempted to use all manner of over-the-counter treatments to provide comfort. But you could be putting your child's health at risk if you don't read the medicine label carefully. Make sure especially that you aren't inadvertently harming your child by handing out too much of one particular ingredient. You might administer the recommended dose of paracetamol tablets, for instance, but not notice that the cough medicine you're also providing contains the same drug. Too much paracetamol can cause liver damage. So always check the small print on the packaging.

Measure medicines accurately

Surveys have discovered that many people don't know how

to measure liquid medicines properly. Too often, they use a normal teaspoon, which doesn't deliver the full 5ml of liquid. So save that teaspoon for stirring hot drinks and use a medicine spoon or syringe instead.

Keep taking the tablets

A report that analysed 21 studies found that people who take their medicine as prescribed have a lower risk of dying within a specified time period than those who don't take it or take it irregularly. Don't rely on doctors to remind you how important it is to follow their prescriptions. Many surveys have shown medical practitioners are notoriously bad when it comes to counselling their patients. They hardly ever mention the most important point about any prescribed drug – that if you don't take it, it definitely won't do you any good.

Skip paracetamol

Does your doctor still recommend paracetamol to numb the pain of arthritis? Then ask for an alternative, such as ibuprofen, or maybe cut out the drugs and try some form of exercise. A major study published in the Archives of Internal Medicine has found that paracetamol, an ingredient in many painkillers, often worked no better than a placebo, or dummy pill. Plus, in large doses it can cause kidney and liver damage.

THE BEST OF BOTH WORLDS? In the near future you may have a third option beyond just generic and brand-name drugs. Pharmaceutical giants such as Eli Lilly, Pfizer and Abbott Labs are getting into the generic-drug business with so-called 'branded generics'. These medications are an appealing compromise for many who desire a trusted brand at a more affordable price. They are primarily being marketed in Europe and Asia at the moment.

Assess
alternative therapies

In a classic case of 'the grass is always greener', Western consumers are turning toward Eastern and alternative health remedies (the UK spends more than £350 million a year on natural remedies and health supplies), while our counterparts around the world continue to envy Western medical advances. Who's right? Probably both, but until the two schools merge, here's how to weigh your options.

Remember these two important things

Manufacturers of dietary supplements do not have to prove the safety or efficacy of their products before selling them (and 'natural' doesn't mean 'safe'). There is also no statutory regulation of any complementary and alternative medicine (CAM) practitioners except chiropractors, osteopaths and those practising herbal medicine.

But there are some useful resources...

First, there's the American National Centre for Complementary and Alternative Medicine. It's a clearinghouse for education and research and its excellent website (nccam.nih.gov) is a must when considering any unconventional treatment. It offers background on specific therapies and highlights new research. Then, in the UK, the Government-supported Complementary and Natural Healthcare Council (cnhc.org.uk) offers information on finding a reliable therapist and has a voluntary register of practitioners that the public can consult.

Watch for red-flag words

Miracle cure, revolutionary discovery, secret ingredient, ancient remedy, cure-all, purify, detoxify, energise... These are all descriptions designed to excite rather than inform. When you see any of them on a website or advertisement, beware. It's even worse if 'operators are standing by to take your order on this special one-time offer'.

Consider the cost

Although you can sometimes get CAM therapies like acupuncture, homeopathy and chiropractic on the NHS, most have to be paid for and some are pretty expensive.

Let your doctor be your guide

Although GPs are conventionally trained, most are familiar with alternative therapies and can help assess the relative risks and benefits (and maybe even the practitioner or manufacturer). More important, your doctor will warn you if a supplement could interact with what you're already taking. For instance, taking ginkgo biloba if you're already on Warfarin could raise your risk of internal bleeding, since both are blood thinners.

Consider integrating

If you're dissatisfied with your current mode of treatment but still want to explore CAM therapies with a safety net, consider integrative medicine. Many GPs now offer complementary therapies so check with yours to see if your doctor or someone else in the practice does.

YOU: A GUINEA PIG One way to be on the cusp of alternative healthcare is to participate in a clinical trial. These are research studies in which specific therapies are evaluated. The National Centre for Complementary and Alternative Medicine in the US maintains a database of trials, including ones recruiting volunteers in the UK, where you can see what's upcoming and how you can register. Although there are risks involved (after all, these treatments are experimental), depending on where you're at in the management of your condition, it might be worthwhile. For more information, visit nccam.nih.gov/research/clinicaltrials/factsheet.

Buy medicine
online safely

Online shopping is fun, convenient and economical, but buying pills on the internet is very different to purchasing a jacket from Boden. There are thousands of online-pharmacy websites but the Government's Medicines and Healthcare Products Regulatory Agency can only monitor and, if necessary, take action against British ones. And as we know the worldwide web is, well... worldwide. This means if you're not careful about buying drugs online, the health of you and your family could be in jeopardy.

Click off the 'no prescription necessary' sites

No matter how tempting it may be to order drugs such as Viagra without the embarrassment of seeing a doctor, if an online seller doesn't require a prescription, there's a good chance the pills you receive (if you get them at all) will be counterfeit, improperly formulated or expired. Many reputable web-based pharmacies have an online doctor who can issue prescriptions anyway.

Check the hit list

All pharmacies in Great Britain, including online operations, must be registered with the General Pharmaceutical Council (GPhC). Consult the register at pharmacyregulation.org before buying any meds on the web. Or just look for the Green Cross logo and GPhC registration number on the pharmacy's home page, though this is voluntary. Also check that the name of the owner and the address of the business are given. Your healthcare provider may also be able to recommend reputable online services, especially now that you can submit NHS as well as private prescriptions to some virtual pharmacies.

Beware of going abroad

Recent research from the Co-Operative Pharmacy found that over a third of internet shoppers bought drugs from the US and one in eight sourced meds from Eastern Europe. Whether or not they're prescription medicines, there's no guarantee that they meet UK regulatory and quality standards unless they are supplied by a registered UK-based pharmacy. So despite how trustworthy these sites appear to be, remember that you have no legal recourse if their products harm you.

Compare prices

Don't assume you always get the best deal online. By the time you pay for shipping and handling or next-day delivery, your savings may not be that substantial. It may pay you to develop a relationship with a local pharmacist instead. Some of the big chains now have their own online operations, allowing you to manage your NHS prescription from the comfort of your home.

Watch the weather forecast

Drugs can lose their potency long before the expiration date if exposed to oxygen, heat, light or humidity. Check if your meds have temperature recommendations on their labels. If so, either ask your online supplier to ship accordingly or buy locally.

PILLS FOR PETS If you have pets, you know how expensive keeping them healthy can get, but ordering medications over the internet carries the same risks for them as it does for you. The Government's Veterinary Medicines Directorate (VMD) has a voluntary accreditation scheme for internet retailers of pet meds in the UK. Websites that dispense and supply drugs for pets are asked to display a logo. Your own vet will issue you with a prescription you can use on the net, though he'll make a charge for it, so bear that in mind when considering price.

Avoid
medical errors

You are more likely to die from a medical error than from cancer or a car crash. Even the Department of Health's estimates suggest that there are a staggering 850,000 medical accidents each year in English hospitals. Healthcare officials are working to reduce these figures, but there are also ways you, as a patient, can help. Here are the top ten recommendations, based on the National Patient Safety Agency's 'Top 10 tips for Safer Patients'.

1

Find out all you can about your treatment. Ask questions and gather information from patient groups and the internet. Research shows that people who are involved with their care tend to get better results.

2

Ask your doctor to explain all the options for treatment that are open to you, including any potential risks.

3

If you're not quite sure what a doctor or nurse is saying, ask them to repeat it. If you don't understand, ask them to explain any medical terms in everyday language.

4

If you're allergic to anything or have reacted badly to a medicine or an anaesthetic in the past, make sure you tell everyone who's treating you: doctors, nurses, the anaesthetist – if you're having an operation – and the pharmacist.

5

If you or your child are going to have an operation, check that all the details on the consent form are correct before you sign it.

6

Always read the instructions on medicines. Check that you understand why you're taking something, how to take it and for how long. Note any possible side effects and what to do if they occur. Ask if it is safe to take with other medicines or dietary supplements and what foods or activities to avoid.

> *'It is a mathematical fact that 50 per cent of all doctors graduate in the bottom half of their class.'*
>
> – Anonymous

7

If a family member or friend needs treatment and has difficulty communicating or understanding what is happening, go along too, to help to explain and ask questions.

8

When in hospital, make sure that every member of your healthcare team has accurate information about you, the medicines you are taking and the treatment or operation you're in for.

9

If you're pregnant, or think you might be, make sure you tell the doctor, nurse or radiographer before you have an X-ray, scan or any radiation treatment.

10

Always ask doctors, nurses, ward staff, porters and anyone else who is about to touch you or any equipment you're using, if they've washed their hands.

Shop like a
nutritionist

Imagine if you were able to look over the shoulder of a mechanic diagnosing car trouble or assist a master chef preparing dinner for six. You'd learn loads because experts like these know all the tricks. So we decided to shadow some nutritionists on a trip to the supermarket. Here are their secrets for getting in, getting out and most importantly, getting you healthy.

Eat something beforehand

Never go shopping on an empty stomach. You're more likely to splash out on biscuits and crisps if you're hungry. No matter how pure your intentions, you'll undoubtedly glaze over, succumb to temptation and pile lots of unhealthy food into your trolley. Nutritionists always shop after meals.

Come with a plan

The experts never wing it. They devise a healthy meal plan ahead of time and make a list of all the necessary ingredients. This keeps them focused.

Hire a surrogate shopper

Believe it or not, some nutritionists don't shop. Instead, they order online and get their groceries delivered. Although this can cost extra, they find it actually saves money (and time) because they don't buy items on impulse. Alternatively, one nutritionist gets her husband or son to do the shopping. This strategy is based on a Food Marketing Institute survey that concluded men are more likely than women to stick to a shopping list. (Warning: this approach does not work with men in the tools department at B&Q.)

Grab a smaller trolley

This trick employs the same psychology as eating from smaller dinner plates or bowls when you're trying to lose weight. With limited space you won't overbuy and, later, overeat.

Patrol the perimeter first

Traditionally, the outer supermarket aisles are where the freshest, most healthy foods are located – meats, fish, fruits, dairy, vegetables... Nutritionists make the bulk of their buys here.

Make quick turns and look up and down

When they must delve into the middle of the store, nutritionists usually ignore the displays at the heads of the aisles and almost everything at eye level. This is where you typically find crisps, biscuits, soft drinks and other less nutritious (but highly profitable) items.

WANT NOT, WASTE NOT

12 » Per cent of a typical grocery order that people don't eat and eventually throw away.

Look for short ingredient lists

To keep from getting bogged down reading labels, nutritionists often buy the brand with the fewest ingredients. These are generally the least processed and thus are more natural and better for you. (For more label-reading tips, see page 22.)

Know your weaknesses

Buy smart, and be realistic. Even nutritionists like the occasional treat. Include some healthy snack foods and special treats on your shopping list. And remember to add some healthy convenience foods, such as cut-up, bagged fresh vegetables or lower-calorie and lower-sodium frozen foods.

Know when to
see a doctor

Most men would rather tough it out, women are often too busy, and the dog and cat generally prefer to just lick it. Sometimes, though, seeing a doctor is what you need to do, and pronto. Here's how to know when you've crossed that line.

» Ankle injury
Pain and swelling doesn't subside after a few days.

» Backache
Persistent and disabling.

» Bleeding
Any blood coming from any place you've never seen it before.

» Bug bite
Bull's-eye-type rash with a red centre and ring, accompanied by flulike symptoms and joint pain, especially if you live in an area where Lyme disease (spread to humans by ticks) is prevalent.

» Chest discomfort
Pressure or pain in the middle of the chest, with shortness of breath, nausea, cold sweats or tingling in the arms.

» Cold
Persists more than 10 days or is accompanied by high fever, significantly swollen glands or severe sinus pain.

» Constipation
Lasts more than two weeks and is generally unresponsive to laxatives or is accompanied by intense abdominal/rectal pain.

» Cough

Produces pinkish or greenish yellow phlegm, plus difficulty breathing and fever.

» Earache

Persists more than a day, with pain and discharge.

» Fever

Lasts more than three days or is higher than 39°C (103°F).

» Headache

Sudden, severe or accompanied by confusion, fainting, dizziness, slurred speech, blurred vision, nausea, high fever or numbness.

» Lumps

Anything that pops up anywhere without an identifiable cause, whether it hurts or not.

» Nausea

Vomiting lasts more than two days, inability to drink for 24 hours, history of heart disease or diabetes.

» Pain

Anything unusual, severe or stubborn.

» Peeing

If the urge becomes frequent, the process is painful or if the urine has a reddish tinge not attributable to diet or medication.

» Postnatal sadness

Baby blues lasting longer than two weeks and accompanied by withdrawal, mood swings or thoughts of harming the infant.

» Snoring

Regularly waking up with a choking snort that leaves you breathless, plus excessive daytime drowsiness.

» Sore throat

Unusually severe, lasting longer than a week, or is joined by fever, difficulty breathing or blood-tinged saliva.

» Spots

Any noticeable change to the shape, colour or size of a mole, freckle or other patch of skin.

» Stress

When it results in a significant decline of work/school performance, excess anxiety, misuse of alcohol/drugs, irrational fears, changes in sleeping/eating habits, sustained withdrawal or suicidal thoughts.

» Weight loss

Any significant drop not resulting from a change in diet, exercise or illness.

GET IN LINE

18 ‣ Per cent of GP consultations are about minor ailments that could have been self-managed by the patient or dealt with by a trip to a pharmacist.

51.4 million ‣ Number of GP consultations that 18 per cent figure equates to.

£1.5 billion ‣ Amount of money all those unnecessary visits cost the taxpayers.

Source: Royal Pharmaceutical Society

Best ③0 minute workout:
Run/walk

Nothing beats running for a quick, thorough, cardiovascular workout. Plus, it burns lots of calories, tones leg muscles and is so simple and convenient it can be done anywhere. But if you're out of shape or new to running, don't just put on your shoes and take off for half an hour. That'll be too exhausting, and you could injure yourself in the process. Instead, after checking with your doctor, build up to the activity by following this 30-minute programme from *Runner's World* magazine. In just seven short weeks you'll be running the entire time, and a whole new world of health and fitness will open up.

▸▸ *The Code*
   W = Walk   m = minutes
   R = Run   x = times (as in repeat 6x)

▸▸ *The Frequency*
   Do each workout four times per week (i.e., Monday, Wednesday, Friday and Saturday). On other days either walk for 30 minutes (Tuesday and Thursday) or rest entirely (Sunday). As far as pace, maintain what's comfortably challenging.

▸▸ *The Plan*

   Week 1: Walk for 30 minutes

   Week 2: 4mW/1mR, 6x = (6 total minutes of running)

   Week 3: 2mW/1mR, 10x = (10 total minutes of running)

   Week 4: 1mR/1mW, 15x = (15 total minutes of running)

   Week 5: 2mR/1mW, 10x = (20 total minutes of running)

   Week 6: 4mR/1mW, 6x = (24 total minutes of running)

   Week 7: Run for 30 minutes

Find the right diet for you

Search 'diet books' on Amazon and you'll find 46,517 options. Eat baby food to lose weight! Oops, didn't work? Try these doctor-endorsed biscuits instead! No, no, the answer is caveman cuisine! Wait, our mistake. Listen to Zoe Ball, Alicia Silverstone or Martine McCutcheon... If you're confused, overwhelmed, or if it feels like you've personally tried every one of these 46,517 plans and still don't have the body you want, it's time to regroup.

Get your terms straight

One of the reasons this country is getting fatter is because most people don't understand the meaning of the word 'diet.'

POPULAR DEFINITION	PROPER DEFINITION
Short term	Long term
Fad	Lifestyle
Celebrity	Reality
Elimination	Moderation
Losing weight	Staying healthy

See the difference? A diet shouldn't be a fast fix; it should be a life plan. To tell one from the other is a simple matter of asking, Can I eat this way for the rest of my life? If the answer is no, don't even try it.

Simplify the science

A study reported in the *New England Journal of Medicine* tracked 811 overweight adults on a variety of low-carb, low-fat, high-protein diets. Most of the diets had clever-sounding theories and narrow research findings behind them that, when read in isolation, sounded awfully convincing. Several were detailed in bestselling books. And yet, after two years no single diet emerged as the best. 'The real key,' says J. Graham Thomas at the Weight Control and Diabetes Research Centre in the US, 'is energy balance. To lose weight you must burn more energy than you eat, and for weight maintenance the two must be in balance.' You don't need a magic diet to accomplish this; you just need the knowledge and resolve to ensure that activity cancels out calories every day.

Understand your daily cycle

So how do you begin to get a grip on daily energy balance? Keeping a daily food and exercise diary can help reveal patterns such as when you overeat. But a convenient tool that's worked for many is a mobile phone app such as FatSecret. It's a daily calorie and exercise tracker that you can download for free (visit fatsecret.co.uk to learn more). Using it over time imparts a better sense of how nutrition and activity work together. Indeed, in an ongoing study of 6,000 people who have lost at least 13kg and kept it off for a year or more, a key to success is daily self-monitoring just like that. 'These people know on a daily basis whether they're heading in the right direction or not,' explains Thomas. 'Tracking food intake, weight and physical activity lets them make instant adjustments.'

HOW FAD DIETS MAKE YOU FAT Your body can't tell the difference between dieting and starving. When you significantly cut calories for an extended period, it automatically lowers its metabolism to conserve energy and protect its existence. But when you can no longer endure the crazy diet you're on and food reappears, metabolism stays low and the additional calories are stored as fat in anticipation of the next 'famine'.

Although it's a remarkably efficient system for ensuring the continuation of the species, it condemns those who repeatedly experience it to even higher weights and body-fat percentages. This is the curse of 'weight cycling' or 'yo-yo dieting'. To avoid it, make sure any weight-loss programme you embark on is slow, sustainable and accompanied by exercise.

Stay calm in an MRI

Some medical sounds scare the hell out of us. There's the high-pitched whirr of a dentist's drill, the flat-line whine of an EKG and perhaps worst of all, that incessant banging during an MRI. While there's not much you can do about the first two, there are plenty of ways to make an MRI more bearable.

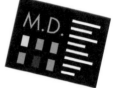

Understand what's happening
As with anything, the more information you have, the less anxious you'll be. MRI stands for Magnetic Resonance Imaging. As you remain motionless in the scanner, radio waves in a magnetic field produce detailed images of your insides. The process is safer and more precise than X-rays, and that banging noise is the normal sound of the scanner's gradient coils and magnetic fields at work.

Ask about an open MRI
Because of their tunnel-like design, traditional closed scanners can trigger claustrophobia and panic attacks. Newer, open scanners aren't as confining and reduce those risks. But not all centres have them, and depending on what you're getting done, traditional types may be more accurate. If you are claustrophobic, you could ask for a mild sedative to help you relax. Talk to your GP or consultant about this well in advance of having the scan. If you do decide to have a sedative, you will need to arrange for someone to drive you home afterwards.

Arrange for a health buddy
It always helps to have a hand to hold, so a friend or family member may be allowed to stay in the room with you. Children can usually have a parent with them. Anyone who stays with you will be asked whether they have a pacemaker or any other metal objects in their body.

Empty your bladder

Since you'll have to remain motionless for up to an hour, never load up on coffee or other liquids before a scan.

Listen to your favourite tracks

You may be surprised at how noisy an MRI scanner is when it's in operation. Some radiographers will have a music system so you can take a CD along to help you to relax and give you something to focus on.

Don't open your eyes

That's when many people start losing it, especially in a closed unit, so keep your eyes closed. You may be offered eye pads or gel eye masks or be able to take your own along.

BREATHE LIKE THIS Anxiety builds when you're not breathing enough. This raises the heart rate, deprives the brain of oxygen (essential for rational thought) and makes you feel out of control. To keep this from happening during an MRI, do this:

1. *Exhale thoroughly.*

2. *Inhale through your nose for 3 seconds.*

3. *Purse your lips and exhale to a count of 10 (or however long you can) while letting your cheeks puff out. Get every last bit of air out.*

4. *Repeat until you're calm.*

The long exhalation ensures that the next inhalation is automatically deeper, explains Al Lee, co-author of *Perfect Breathing*. This counters the tendency to take short, shallow breaths when you're scared. Practice this exercise beforehand.

Handle an overseas
health emergency

True story. We were on a cruise in the South Pacific when a passenger fell gravely ill. He was taken to a hospital at the next port, but because he needed a blood transfusion and conditions there were deplorable, his wife had him airlifted to New Zealand. Fortunately, he survived, but the £30,000 medical bill nearly killed him. Which goes to prove, Montezuma's revenge is the least of your worries when travelling abroad. Be prepared.

Check your health coverage

If you're travelling in the European Economic Area (EEA), the European Health Insurance Card (EHIC) replaced the old E111 in 2006. It's free and you can apply online at ehic.org.uk. But it's not an alternative to travel insurance and won't cover any private medical healthcare or costs such as mountain rescue in ski resorts, being flown back to the UK or lost or stolen property, so you'll still need to buy travel insurance for full coverage.

Good coverage

Travel insurance will cover medical costs that the EHIC will not, such as transporting you to the nearest medical centre for appropriate care, paying for your return journey if illness delays you or covering your personal contributions towards treatment. You will also receive cover for non-medical emergencies, such as replacing stolen possessions or a lost passport. Your policy will vary according to your destination, but cover generally starts at just a few pounds and could save you thousands of pounds.

Be your own mobile medical file

To speed diagnosis and treatment in a foreign land, keep all your vital health information handy (for example, blood type, allergies, medications, pre-existing conditions). Your doctor's office can supply the information. Another option is a service such as MedicAlert (medicalert.org.uk), a charity providing a life-saving identification system, which has a medical information service.

Learn the 999 equivalent

Many people assume 999 works internationally, but it doesn't. In the USA and Canada , for instance, the emergency services number is 911, and throughout the European Union 112. Look up the number for your destination before you leave (it will usually be listed in your guide book) and programme it into your phone.

When in doubt, call the embassy

The Foreign & Commonweath Office (FCO) maintains embassies, high commissions and diplomatic services in most major cities and countries. They're your safety net when travelling abroad. Find contact information for each, as well as travel advice and information by country, at fco.gov.uk.

FOR NEXT TIME Before you go away again, follow these tips to lower your risk of a health emergency abroad:

▸▸ **Get your teeth checked:** consider having a dental check-up before you go, especially if you are going on a long trip

▸▸ **Get your jabs:** find out what vaccinations are required at www.cdc.gov/travel. Your GP will advise on vaccination schedules.

▸▸ **Get it in writing:** take a letter from your GP about any pre-existing medical conditions. Get this translated or find someone to act as a translator if you cannot find an English-speaking doctor.

Make these health moves in your 40s

What	When
Routine checks/exams	
Complete physical	Every 5 years
Blood pressure	Every 5 years *(more frequently if at risk)*
Cholesterol	Every 5 years *(more frequently if at risk)*
Blood glucose	Every 5 years *(annually for those who are overweight or have a family history of Type 1 diabetes)*
Eyesight	Every 2 years
Teeth	At least every 2 years *(seek guidance from your dentist)*
Body mass index (BMI)	Every 6 months
Testicular cancer	Monthly self-examination
Breast cancer/mammogram	Monthly self-examination, first mammogram between 47 and 50
Cervical smear	Every 3 years

For many this is the wake-up decade. The number on the bathroom scale creeps up, a routine medical test comes back positive or a family member or friend is unexpectedly hospitalised. The good news is, we're all remarkably resilient. If your health hasn't been a priority through the first half of life, now is the time to make your comeback.

Inoculations

Various	If missed in prior decades (see page 42)

General

Go low-impact.	Hang up the running shoes and switch to joint-friendly workouts.
Adopt a dog.	Pets lower blood pressure.
Prioritise happiness.	Risk of depression is high.
Eat smarter.	Metabolism is still declining.
Get more calcium/vitamin D.	It boosts bone health, especially for women.

Assess the health of
your workplace

Each of us gets sick of working every now and then. But if your symptoms go beyond ordinary stress to actual feelings of illness, it's time to conduct a thorough job review.

Is anyone else feeling this way?
Ask your work colleagues. If others are experiencing headaches, burning eyes, respiratory problems, itching, dizziness, nausea, chronic fatigue or other discomforts that coincide with the workday, it may be a case of Sick Building Syndrome. This can stem from inadequate ventilation or chemical/biological contaminants. Take your evidence to HR or the boss, but couch your complaint in terms of lowered productivity and sick days.

Are you sitting comfortably?
Sit all the way back in your chair or select a back cushion that provides the right support. Providing adequate lumbar support to reduce stress to your lower back is important, as is making sure your feet rest firmly on the floor; use a footrest if they don't. Adjust the height of your chair so your upper arms are relaxed at your sides and your elbows at even height with your keyboard.

Can I hear myself think?
A noisy work environment, where you must raise your voice to be heard, makes heart trouble three to four times more likely. It raises diastolic blood pressure, which means arteries never relax between heartbeats and blood flow is chronically constricted. If possible, wear noise-cancelling headphones or earplugs.

Am I sitting down all day?
Doing so for more than six hours per day raises your chance of dying by 18 per cent (for men) and 37 per cent (for women)

compared with those who sit less than three hours daily. Frequent breaks help, but what's even better is raising your work station. Standing burns calories, fights disease and improves concentration and productivity.

Do others share my workspace?
If your desk or cubicle isn't really *your* desk or cubicle, start every shift by disinfecting with antibacterial wipes the desk, keyboard, phone, armrests and anything else you touch.

Do I have access to fresh air and natural light?
If not, turn off the overhead fluorescents (a possible headache trigger) and open the window when possible. If you're trapped, decorate your workspace with peace lily, Gerbera daisies, chrysanthemums or bamboo palms. In a NASA study these were among the best indoor plants at filtering formaldehyde, benzene and trichloroethylene from the air. These chemicals can be generated by paint, carpeting and machinery.

Do I have a company phone?
It may seem like a bonus, but if your boss considers it his 24/7 hotline to you, it can blur boundaries between home and work, leaving you stressed and your health compromised. Turn it off and return calls when *you're* available.

JUST HOW CRAZED ARE YOU AT WORK? Here's an easy way to tell: instead of a watch, wear a heart-rate monitor. It'll supply an ongoing display of the stress of your workday. You can even set the upper-limit alarm to quietly beep when your pulse rises above a certain point. Over time you'll learn who and what sets you off and, more importantly, how to step back, take a deep breath and actually lower your pulse.

Manage an
elderly parent

Around 2.8 million British adults over the age of 50 are caring for elderly parents. What's ironic is that in their well-intentioned efforts to safeguard Mum and Dad's health, they're often compromising their own. High numbers report stress, anxiety or depression, and studies also link the process to weight gain and lower overall levels of self-care. If you're doing this job now or anticipating it in the near future, here's how to minimise the wear-and-tear.

Get Grandma wired
Communication is the key to managing this life stage, and nothing makes it easier than the internet. Email, video chat, photo sharing, Google and the old standby Solitaire can all help the elderly feel less alone. Be sure to consider tablet devices such as the Apple iPad. Many seniors prefer these over traditional computers and even mobile phones, because of their size and ease of use.

Work out the legal stuff
End-of-life issues are complicated, and laws change, so consult a solicitor personally about what to set up in advance. These include living wills, powers of attorney, organ donation and do-not-resuscitate orders. Granted, these are uncomfortable discussions to have, but a solicitor will facilitate them and ensure there are no legal hassles.

Become a health buddy
Join your mum for medical check-ups (or at least talk to her doctor or nurse by phone afterwards) to be sure nothing is overlooked. Being fully informed will help ease your worry and better prepare you to take action when necessary. In addition,

monitor her medication for side effects and use reliable sources on the internet to help stay on top of her conditions (websites ending in .org, .gov and .edu are most trustworthy). Elderly people tend to have blind faith in doctors and healthcare. You need to be their watchdog.

Muster plenty of troops

Statistics show that most caregivers are ill-prepared for their role and provide care with little or no support. There are three basic resources to tap:

1. *Family: if you have siblings in the area, divide the duties. Ask your spouse or the grandkids to help, too. Having everyone pitch in will ease the burden while making Grandpa feel well loved.*

2. *Neighbours: ask your Facebook friends if they know anyone in the area who'd be willing to pick up groceries or drive Mum to the hairdressers when you can't. There are lots of people out there happy to do good deeds.*

3. *Public services: some local councils offer free programmes or services for the elderly or support for carers. Age UK (ageuk.org.uk) offers free information and advice for the elderly about benefits, travel, health, activities and more. If you need support, Carers Direct at nhs.uk/carersdirect offers free advice (0808 802 0202) or can put you in touch with services for carers near you.*

Keep this in mind

Some of the best advice we ever got about coping with the challenges of caring for the elderly comes from educator Angela Lunde at the Mayo Clinic. 'Blame the disease, not the person, when caregiving gets frustrating,' she says. By realising it's not your mum or dad's fault, you'll be better able to treat them (and yourself) with compassion.

{ What can I do to help my parents and family be }
more healthy?

Is genetic testing for you?

Genetic testing is possible for about 2,000 diseases, and more tests are being refined daily. No doubt it'll play a large role in future prevention, diagnosis and treatment. But for now it's much less black and white than it seems. Not only is the science still developing, but there are also moral, ethical and psychological issues involved. Although it's tempting to peek at your DNA, especially since home test kits are now available, there are important questions to ask before moving forwards.

Why are you considering it?

Curiosity alone shouldn't be the driver. Genetic testing is best done under a doctor's supervision when 1) there's a strong first-degree family history of a disease, 2) there's a risk of a child acquiring a serious affliction, or 3) you have symptoms requiring further diagnosis.

What are you looking for?

If it's a predisposition to cystic fibrosis; sickle cell anemia; or breast, ovarian or colon cancer, genetic testing is more dependable. But for the vast majority of diseases, the genetic link is either less clear or not established. For example, it's estimated that 90 to 95 per cent of all cancers *don't* have an inherited component that strongly affects risk.

Can you afford it?

Any genetic test deemed necessary by your doctor will be paid for by the NHS. More wide-ranging personal genomics tests which analyse a person's DNA and provide risk estimates of various diseases are expensive, ranging from about £350 up to many thousands of pounds.

How vital is your privacy?

A moratorium agreed by the Association of British Insurers and the Department of Health means that an adverse genetic test result will not affect a person's ability to take out any insurance, with the exception of life insurance of over £500,000. Anti-discrimination laws covered by the Equality Act of 2010 prevent any employment decision being made because of genetic tests. But in these days of information proliferation and account hacking, could you cope if something leaked out?

Can you handle the verdict?

Learning you're carrying a potentially deadly gene that you may have passed along to your children is some heavy psychological baggage. A positive result doesn't guarantee development of disease, but it does assure some degree of worry, probably for the rest of your life.

Will you act on the results?

If you'll use a positive result as an impetus to make meaningful lifestyle changes, then knowledge is power. But if you're more likely to do nothing or, worse, forgo prevention because you think a negative result is ironclad protection (which it's not), then knowing you're at risk may actually increase your risk.

Are you enough of an expert to make this decision?

Most people aren't. In fact, many doctors don't fully appreciate all the implications of genetic testing. The smartest move if you're serious about moving forward is to meet with a genetic counsellor. These specialists will help you answer all the questions we just raised. Your GP may refer you to a genetics service, particularly if your family has a genetic condition.

Finding
solutions

When it comes to repairing some health issues and insulating yourself against others, there's a lot you can do on your own. In that respect, this section is your B&Q – the land of the personal health handyman. From soothing your various aches and pains to decreasing your risk of diabetes and cancer, each chapter is a separate, well-stocked aisle.

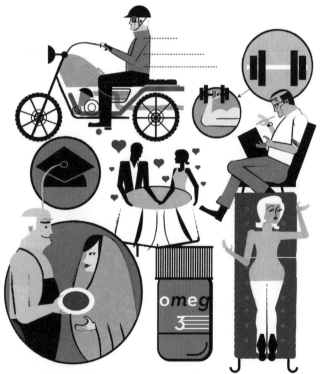

Turn off a
headache

Doctors can replace entire hearts and hips, but when it comes to something as everyday as a headache, they're still often perplexed. That's because there are more than 150 different types, each with unique symptoms, severities and causes that range from anxiety to allergies, hypertension to hormones, ice cream to orgasms. When it seems like Charlie Watts is drumming in your head, here's how to stop him.

Have a cup of coffee and two ibuprofen gel caps
Studies point to this combo as providing the fastest and longest-lasting relief from most headaches. The caffeine apparently speeds delivery of the medication, while also shrinking swollen blood vessels in the head. For more debilitating migraines the combination of, for example, paracetamol, codeine and buclizine (Migraleve) or aspirin and metoclopramide (Migramax) appears to work better.

Become a headhunter
To find the source of your hurt, start keeping a headache journal. This is a simple matter of recording what you were doing in the hours before the pain struck. Meals, mood, time of day, location – note it all, along with how the headache feels and where it's located (temples, sinus, behind the eye, forehead, neck and so on). Eventually, certain patterns may emerge that point to specific triggers, which can then be avoided.

Stay away from Tyra
Roughly 20 per cent of migraine headaches are diet-induced, and it's not just MSG and alcohol that are responsible. A naturally occurring amino acid called tyramine is often to

blame. It's especially concentrated in foods that are aged, dried, fermented or stored for long periods. Cheese, processed meat, nuts, red wine and even gherkins can be instigators.

Switch off the light

Certain types of flickering or glaring light from fluorescent bulbs, computer monitors, TV screens and even the sun (in snow or beach conditions) can cause headaches. To minimise the effects, turn off overhead office lighting (or counter it with incandescent table lamps), install antiglare screens and wear polarised sunglasses outdoors.

See a specialist

The previous steps often help, but if not, don't suffer in silence. A headache, unless its source is the other family members living in your home, does not have to be chronic. Beyond over-the-counters and home remedies, there is expert help available in the form of migraine clinics and neurologists. There are even some interesting treatments, including Botox facial injections, which promise to make you feel *and* look better!

THE BIG THREE There are three general categories of headaches: tension, migraine and cluster. *Tension headaches* are the most common. They're caused by anxiety, fatigue or a stressful environment and make your head feel like it's being crushed in a vice. *Migraine headaches* are more intense, characterised by throbbing pain, nausea and hypersensitivity to light and noise. They have assorted triggers, including food, hormones and weather. *Cluster headaches* are often the most continuously painful, centring on one side of the head or behind an eye. As their name implies, these don't last long (30 to 45 minutes) but recur throughout the day.

Stop the snoring

If your partner sounds like a '69 Mustang with an open throttle when he's 'sleeping', then your relationship (and your health) are in serious trouble. Having your rest routinely disturbed by a chronic snorer can lead to arguments, lower libido, resentment, separate bedrooms and even divorce. Poor sleep is also linked to high blood pressure, stroke and diabetes. Since it's often difficult to get someone to admit to a snoring problem, let alone see a specialist, here are some sneaky ways you can try to fix it.

Move up last call
Snoring is caused by the vibration of loose throat tissue as air passes over it. Alcohol consumption further relaxes throat muscles and thereby compounds the tendency to snore. Make last orders at least two hours before lights out.

Raise the head of the bed
To keep his tongue from flopping back over his airway (hey, you married him), put a 10-cm brick or sturdy block under each leg at the head of the bed. As a beauty bonus for you, it will reduce facial blood pooling and eye puffiness. It also helps counteract heartburn.

Promote healthy eating
A poor diet not only promotes obesity, which fattens throat tissue and narrows air passages, it can also cause acid reflux, which further inflames that area.

Decongest the area
Allergies and colds are another common cause of snoring. Offer a decongestant before bed or a nasal strip such as Breathe Right or Snoreeze, which helps to keep your nostrils open while you are sleeping.

Finding solutions

Hide the sleeping pills

If your mate relies on medication to sleep, he may unwittingly be compounding the problem. Such drugs generally work by depressing the central nervous system and further relaxing throat muscles.

Get off his back

Because snoring is compounded by sleeping face up, try duct-taping or sewing a golf ball to the back of his pyjama top. This will keep him on his side.

Spark an interest in music

According to a *British Medical Journal* study, regularly playing a didgeridoo (a traditional Australian wind instrument) reduces snoring by toning throat muscles. If it turns out the sound of him playing a didgeridoo is even worse than the snoring itself, encourage singing instead. Twenty minutes per day of certain vocal exercises, such as la-la-la and ma-ma-ma, may have the same effect another report states.

Get help if you hear this...

Although these home remedies are often effective, if your partner frequently awakens with a start from his snores or it seems as if his breathing is interrupted, take him to a doctor immediately. He may have sleep apnoea, a condition that can damage lungs nearly as much as smoking.

RECORD THE RUMBLING If all else fails, put a mobile phone or tape recorder on your bedside cabinet and press the record button the next time you're awakened by the din. Then play it through your stereo system on continuous loop at high volume when your bed partner is trying to have a little quiet time. He'll get the idea. Plus, his doctor can use the recording to diagnose sleep apnoea on his next visit.

Tell if it's impotence
or **anxiety**

What we're really discussing here is the difference between physical and psychological erectile dysfunction (ED). The former results from a specific problem in the body that prevents the penis from getting hard enough for intercourse, while the latter, which is to blame in up to 20 per cent of cases, stems from more elusive mental issues of which boredom can be just one. Since many men find it humiliating to consult a doctor about this, here are a few easy ways to assess if it's a physical problem that requires medical help or a psychological one that could work itself out.

Assess his stress
Anxiety over career, finances, relationships, looks, even kids can distract a man from the task at hand. So if he's been going through a rough patch lately (and drinking more alcohol to cope), then the combination could be what's leaving him limp.

Is he getting enough sleep?
Physically, a lack of sleep can elevate cortisol levels, which also leads to low libido. One study found that men with restless leg syndrome have an increased risk of erectile dysfunction, probably due to low dopamine levels.

Try something fresh
If you've been making love in the same place at the same time in the same way since the beginning of time, reserve an out-of-town room at a romantic B&B and by all means pack the Lady Gaga outfit. If the other guests tell you to keep it down, smile and explain that's exactly the problem you're here to cure.

Peek under the sheets

If he's getting solid erections while asleep, then that's firm evidence any performance problems are psychological.

Inspect his seat

If he took up cycling recently, his saddle might be to blame. Any type of hard or narrow seat that's used for long periods can cause temporary ED by compressing nerves and restricting blood flow. See if function returns after a few days off.

Check the medicine cabinet

Certain antidepressants (Prozac, Zoloft), antihistamines (Benadryl, Dramamine) and nonsteroidal anti-inflammatories (Naproxen) can cause erection problems. If he's started taking any of these lately, consult a doctor about possible alternatives.

See if his heart is still beating

Good erections require good blood flow. That's why impotency can be an early warning sign of heart disease or maybe even diabetes. If your man has a family history of either or has other risk factors (overweight, smoker), treat the lack of a flagpole as a red flag and get medical attention pronto.

ONE PILL MAKES YOU LARGER All those claims made for Viagra, Levitra and Cialis aren't just marketing hype. A study of nearly 8,000 men found all three improved erectile function and sexual satisfaction after six months of treatment. And in case you were wondering, no other vitamin or herbal supplement has that kind of definitive research behind it.

Make these health moves in
your 50s

What

When

Routine checks/exams

Complete physical	Every 5 years
Blood pressure	Every 5 years
Cholesterol	Every 5 years *(more frequently if you or your family have a history of raised cholesterol)*
Blood glucose	Every 5 years *(annually if you are overweight or have a family history of Type 1 diabetes)*
Eyesight	Every 2 years *(more frequently if you are rapidly getting long-sighted)*
Teeth	At least every two years *(seek guidance from your dentist)*
Body mass index (BMI)	Every 6 months
Prostate specific antigen (PSA)	Once *(ask your doctor)*
Flexible-sigmoidoscopy	Once at age 55 to screen for bowel cancer
Bone density	If at risk *(alert your doctor if you have a family history of osteoporosis)*
Mammogram	Every 3 years + monthly breast self-examination.
Cervical smear test	Every 5 years

Traditionally, this is the best decade of life for many men and women. Career and family pressures have eased, and you have more time, money and wisdom to appreciate life. Congratulations, you've arrived. Now make sure an unexpected health problem doesn't trigger a premature departure.

Inoculations

Various	If missed in prior decades (see page 42)

General

Take up yoga.	Restores flexibility/posture/calm.
Manage midlife changes.	If necessary, consult a specialist.
Eat even smarter.	Metabolism is still declining.
Pursue a passion.	It keeps you young.

Prevent diabetes

Unlike heart attack, stroke or cancer, diabetes doesn't sound like a killer. But an estimated 70,000 to 75,000 people with diabetes die in England every year – accounting for about 15 per cent of all deaths. A 2011 report found that up to 24,000 people with diabetes in England die earlier from causes that could have been avoided through better management of their condition. Fortunately, while you can be genetically predisposed to diabetes, it's mostly caused by lifestyle factors. In fact, according to diabetes researcher Richard Béliveau, adopting a healthy lifestyle can prevent up to 90 per cent of Type 2 cases.

Lose 5 to 7 per cent of your weight
That's all the fat you need to shave in order to enjoy a nearly 60 per cent reduction in risk if you also exercise 150 minutes each week, according to a landmark study sponsored by the National Institutes of Health. It's the most significant step you can take to fight diabetes – one with an even greater effect than the popular antidiabetic drug metformin.

Walk 2½ hours per week
Increased physical activity was one of the ways participants in that study reduced their risk of diabetes. It equates to 30 minutes of walking (or other exercise of moderate intensity) five days per week. To stay committed, block off that half hour on your daily schedule as you would any other important appointment.

Eat a big 'brinner'
People who eat breakfast are 35 to 50 per cent less likely to become overweight and develop insulin resistance. For energy balance it also helps to make your first meal of the day your

biggest meal of the day (call it 'brinner'). Too rushed in the morning? Fill your mug with a healthy coffee smoothie. Blend together 1 cup cold, strong-brewed coffee; 1 banana; 1 cup low-fat vanilla yogurt; 1 cup ice; and if desired, one packet of zero-calorie sweetener.

Go low-cal and low-fat

This was the other way those study participants succeeded. Although it's advice you've probably heard (and tried) many times, here are some new ways to make it stick.

▸▸ **Make friends with fibre.** *A diet rich in whole grains, fruits and vegetables can lower your diabetic risk by up to 34 per cent.*

▸▸ **Swear off fizzy drinks.** *Just one a day, whether regular or diet, has been linked to a 44 per cent greater chance of developing metabolic syndrome, a collection of risk factors for diabetes and cardiovascular disease.*

▸▸ **Watch out for the worst fats.** *That would be saturated and trans fat. Both are prevalent in fast food. Eating just two burgers with fries every week can hike up your odds of metabolic syndrome by as much as 50 per cent.*

Be happy

Depression not only makes it less likely you'll exercise and eat well, it also appears to be a stand-alone risk factor for diabetes. In one study it altered body chemistry in ways that raised insulin resistance 23 per cent among women.

THE DIABETES 11 Based on the latest research gathered by the American Diabetes Association, here are the 11 best foods for fighting this disease. They're all rich in calcium, potassium, fibre, magnesium and vitamins A, C and E – the nutrients that appear to pack the most punch. (Note that the ADA recommends getting them through food, not supplements.)

▶▶ Beans

▶▶ Dark leafy greens

▶▶ Citrus fruit

▶▶ Sweet potatoes

▶▶ Berries

▶▶ Tomatoes

▶▶ Fish (high in omega-3 fatty acids, such as salmon)

▶▶ Whole grains

▶▶ Nuts

▶▶ Skimmed milk

▶▶ Fat-free yogurt

PERSONAL NOTES

{ What will I do today to **prevent** diabetes
or heart disease in the future? }

Beat the blues
(without medicine)

These days everybody wants to be happy all the time. But humans just weren't designed to live that way. It's like a holiday. In order to fully appreciate the sweetness of the beach, you need a job that continually gives you a taste of sun and sand. So the key strategy for weathering bad moods is simply realising they're a natural part of life that will ultimately make you feel happier by comparison. That being said, if you tend to feel down more than up, you might have depression, a real disease. Here are some natural solutions for bad moods and their more serious counterpart.

Sweat up a smile

Exercise releases feel-good hormones called endorphins that appear to be even more potent than antidepressants. A Scottish study found that attending exercise classes for 45 minutes twice a week improved the symptoms of people suffering from depression far better than the same amount of time having health talks and discussions.

Make a habit out of breaking habits

Psychologist Douglas Newburg estimates that 99 per cent of most adults' lives are habit and routine. In fact, since the brain is an expensive organ to operate metabolically (meaning, it uses lots of fuel), its tendency is to run on autopilot. But being in a rut like that can get depressing. To break out, try to do one thing differently every day. Shop somewhere new. Listen to another radio station in the car. Over time you'll get addicted to the way these little deviations wake you up and freshen your outlook.

Shift from a fixed to a growth mindset
Many depressed people feel they're imprisoned by their personalities, that they are who they are and there's nothing they can do about it. Wrong. Yes, we have failures and hit obstacles, but we're all works in progress say psychologists. Try viewing your next setback as a learning opportunity rather than as fate.

Fight D with D
Chronic vitamin D deficiency can make you sadder than necessary. To check on yours, ask your doctor to add a vitamin D analysis to your next blood test. If your level is low, eat more D-rich foods or spend additional time in the sunshine (or in a room lit by daylight full spectrum bulbs).

Pet a pet
Sadness often arises from feeling alone and unloved. But pets, since they make you the centre of their universe, instantly solve that. When, for instance, was the last time anyone peed with joy when you came home from work? 'Nuff said.

SWISS MISS FOR BLISS Sometimes all it takes to turn the corner on a dour mood is a single moment of quiet joy. According to Alan Hirsch at the Smell & Taste Treatment Centre and Research Foundation in Chicago, hot chocolate does this best. Not only does the taste of chocolate boost mood because of its deep-seated reward and comfort connotations, in liquid form its smell also tickles olfactory bulbs and compounds these effects.

Check for
skin cancer

Around 11,000 people are diagnosed with melanoma (a type of skin cancer) every year in the UK, according to Cancer Research UK. That's around 30 people every day. Malignant melanoma (the deadliest variety) incidence rates in Britain have more than quadrupled over the last 30 years, and over the last 25 years, rates in Britain have risen faster than any of the top ten cancers in males and females. Unlike most other diseases, however, you don't need any invasive or expensive tests to catch this one early. At least at the outset, you can be your own dermatologist.

Strip for someone
You can't do a thorough job of this yourself, so recruit your spouse or someone you'd like to know better. Take off all your clothes and, in a well-lit room, get them to examine every inch of you. Look for odd-shaped moles or oversized freckles. Include your scalp, between your fingers and toes, and even in those places where the sun rarely goes. (Then, by all means, return the favour.)

Do the ABCD test
Moles should be examined according to the following criteria: asymmetry (does one half match the other?), border irregularity (are the edges jagged?), colour (is it uniform?), and diameter (is it more than 0.5cm wide?). If anything looks suspicious, visit your GP, who will refer you to a specialist if treatment or investigation is necessary.

Look beyond the alphabet
Other warning signs in or around a mole include redness, swelling, itchiness, tenderness, pain, oozing and bleeding. All are signals to consult an expert as well.

Take some photos

If you're at high risk for skin cancer (or just really bored), you can photograph certain moles to better monitor their evolution. If you're under the care of a dermatologist, it might be possible to email them for a quick opinion.

Inspect yourself

Conduct your own amateur investigation every two or three months. Set up a reminder on your phone or in your diary so that you don't forget.

Carry a dermatologist in your pocket

Skin Scanner is an iPhone/iPad app that scans, analyses and then archives your moles. Simply take a clear photograph of the skin lesion and let the app use its technology to gauge whether it's low, medium or high risk. It even comes with a handy alarm so you don't forget to check your moles.

GOOD BOY If your dog is continually sniffing or licking a part of your body, don't shoo him away. He may be trying to tell you something. Some dogs can actually smell cancer and are being used in research labs to do so. If the spot he's concerned with looks suspicious, get it checked (and give him a treat).

Get rid of a **cold**

The common cold is responsible for more doctor visits and job and school absences in the UK than any other illness. The reason colds are so difficult to cure is because more than 200 distinct viruses are to blame. And 20 to 30 per cent of colds have no known cause. To help unclog our healthcare system, here are some tips on unclogging yourself.

Make sure it's a cold
If you have swollen glands, severe sinus pain, a mucus-producing cough and/or high fever, you could have something worse and you *should* consult a doctor. Conversely, if you have a runny nose, itchy eyes and other minor coldlike symptoms that recur frequently or seasonally, you may have allergies. Know thine enemy.

For temporary relief, take this
One of the most popular over-the-counter adult decongestants is Sudafed. While no OTC med will cure a cold, this one is particularly effective at drying up mucus and preventing it from dripping into your throat and lungs, where it can compound the problem. If you prefer a nasal decongestant spray, there are several to choose from including Vicks.

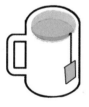

Get into a green routine
Freshly brewed green tea contains a high concentration of EGCG, a natural chemical compound that researchers have found inhibits the replication of the adenovirus cold bug. If swigged at the onset of symptoms, the cold's duration may be shortened.

Have chicken soup (for breakfast)
As the old wives' tale goes, feed that cold. One small study found that a 1,200-calorie breakfast boosts blood levels of

antiviral agents by 450 per cent, which is nothing to sniff at. Some research suggests that having chicken soup for breakfast may reduce the inflammation that causes cold symptoms.

Rest rather than exercise

Although regular exercise strengthens immunity, it's not clear whether it helps chase a cold. People who exercise regularly are less likely to get a cold, some researchers say. A study of 1,000 people found that staying active nearly halved the odds of catching cold viruses and, failing that, made the infection less severe. Because there's a risk of intensifying illness if you exercise too hard with a cold, it's probably smarter to take a few days off. In fact, sleep is the body's preferred way to repair itself.

Play a video game

This is a long shot, but there is some evidence that a short bout of manageable stress, like people typically experience when playing video games, floods the body with disease-fighting proteins. So take one Xbox and call us in the morning.

SUPPLEMENTS FOR SNIFFLES: DO THEY WORK? There are more of them for sale than there are tissues in a box. But are they effective? Here's the verdict from the National Institute of Allergy and Infectious Diseases in the US on the most popular alternative remedies:

▸▸ **Echinacea:** Three big studies found no effect.

▸▸ **Vitamin C:** No clear evidence of any benefit.

▸▸ **Zinc:** May slightly reduce symptoms/duration.

PERSONAL N●TES

{ What are my favourite **home remedies?** }

Quit smoking

Finished. Free. Finally. Getting through the first week is the key. Research shows that within two days of stopping, half of all quitters are lighting up. And by the end of that initial week, two-thirds are back to reaching for a pack. These strategies focus on this crucial period when mental and physical withdrawal symptoms peak and you're most weak.

Put thoughts of cold turkey on ice

The sad fact is that only 4 to 7 per cent of smokers are able to quit without any help, either emotional or medical. That's because smoking isn't just a bad habit; it's an addiction. Admit you need assistance.

Line up someone to lean on

Just as with exercise and weight loss, staying with a commitment is easier if there's someone to support and encourage you. Set a quit date, then schedule an appointment with your doctor, a cognitive behavioural therapist, or a smoking-cessation support group during those first few days. NHS Stop Smoking Services offers support, a list of services in your area and a free hotline (0800 022 4332). One study found that 33 per cent of those who used support services were still smoke-free after 12 months compared to just 5 per cent of those who didn't use any help at all.

Line up some nicotine to wean on

Nicotine-replacement therapy (NRT) supplies the drug you crave in alternative ways, thereby blunting physical withdrawal symptoms. NRTs include chewing gum, lozenges, inhalers, nasal sprays and patches, all with varying degrees of effectiveness. If you're confused by the options, ask your doctor about these as well as prescription medications.

Exercise for five minutes

Whenever the urge hits to go outside for a smoke, take a leisurely five-minute walk. No matter how out of shape you are, you can manage this. Or if there's an exercise bike turned clothes hanger in the house, hop on that for five minutes. The activity will distract you from your craving, reduce stress (a smoking trigger) and counter weight gain (a common side effect of quitting).

Pat yourself on the back frequently

Within 20 minutes of stubbing out that last butt, your heart rate and blood pressure drop. After 12 hours the carbon monoxide in your bloodstream clears. And by the end of the first day, your risk of heart attack is lower. Your circulation is also improving, your sense of taste and smell is returning and your breathing is better (not to mention your breath). Congratulate yourself (repeatedly) on the significant progress you're making. Quitting is the single best thing you can do for your health.

SMOKED MEAT: ANOTHER SMOKING GUN Researchers at the Harvard School of Public Health found that processed meat (smoked, cured, salted and otherwise preserved) contains carcinogens, or potentially cancer-causing compounds. Eating processed meats also raises the risk of heart disease by 42 per cent and Type 2 diabetes by 19 per cent. There is good news, though. This research, which spanned 20 studies and 1.2 million participants, did not find an increased risk from eating *unprocessed* red meat, such as beef, pork and lamb.

PERSONAL NOTES

{ What unhealthy **habits** am I going to try and give up –
and how am I going to do it? }

Extinguish heartburn

Ever hear of hydrochloric acid? It's used to remove rust from steel and dissolve rock during well drilling. It's also the chief ingredient in stomach acid, which explains how it's possible to digest your mother-in-law's Christmas dinner. Sometimes, however, this corrosive acid splashes up into your oesophagus, where it's felt as a burning sensation and can do a lot of damage. If allowed to become chronic, it can even cause cancer. Let's get this under control now.

Gauge the frequency of your burn

For most people heartburn or acid indigestion is an uncomfortable nuisance resulting from an occasional indulgence. But for others it's an ongoing curse stemming from a malfunction in the valve-like muscle linking the stomach with the oesophagus. If your heartburn is frequent (more than twice weekly) and severe, you may have that second condition, which is called gastro-oesophageal reflux disease (GORD).

Flush out the fat

Most people treat their stomachs with less regard than their toilets, throwing in all kinds of junk, then wondering why things keep clogging up. We don't mean to be insensitive to your plumbing woes, but eating smarter (fewer fatty foods/ more fibre), having smaller meals, not lying down for three hours following a meal, and losing weight is the simplest way to reduce episodes of heartburn and GORD. Experiment to find your trigger foods (they're not the same for everybody), and remember that excess kilos put excess pressure on that stomach-oesophagus intersection.

Let Mother Nature be your nurse

There are lots of home remedies for heartburn. Although not long-term solutions, many can provide temporary relief and are worth a try. Chewing gum, for example, produces more saliva, which dilutes acidic backwash. Ginger, either the candied variety or in tea, has been used as a stomach soother for centuries. And although the exact reasons are unclear, a teaspoon of yellow mustard or a couple of almonds after a meal work for some sufferers. The remedy doesn't have to be herbal, either. Some studies have found that elevating the head of your bed 15 to 23cm and sleeping on your left side significantly reduces night-time reflux, as does avoiding sleeping pills.

Call in the pharmacy

Although drugs called PPIs (proton-pump inhibitors), available only on prescription, are very effective, they can shut down stomach-acid production too much if taken for long periods and should be used cautiously. Better to start treatment with milder OTC medications, such as antacids, and then if there's no relief, step up to acid blockers. If you're still suffering, ask your doctor about those PPIs. Most people respond well to treatment with medication but a small number of people with GORD do not respond to medication and need surgery to treat their symptoms.

3 MYTHS DEBUNKED

▸▸ **Heartburn medication should always be taken after a meal:** You may be able to head off heartburn entirely if you take an acid blocker a half hour *before* eating food that normally causes indigestion.

▸▸ **Drinking milk dampens the fire:** It doesn't have any effect on heartburn, and if you're swigging some with a higher fat content, it may actually provoke it.

▸▸ **Heartburn damages the heart:** Although symptoms are sometimes felt in the chest area, stomach acid does not extend to your ticker.

Soothe creaky joints

Do you wake up every morning feeling like the Tin Man in the *Wizard of Oz?* If so, don't believe for a minute that this, like wrinkles and elasticated waistbands, is an inevitable part of growing old. Instead of resigning yourself to analgesics for the rest of your life, here's a well-oiled, medication-free plan for feeling young again.

Make friends with your fascia

Under your skin you wear a suit of interconnected tendons and tissue called fascia. With maturity and mistreatment this suit can begin to feel a few sizes too small, as evidenced by the constricted appearance of so many little old ladies and men. This is all reversible, however, with some appropriate tailoring. First, keep your fascia well hydrated by drinking plenty of water or it will shrivel like a prune. Next, start doing yoga practice to gradually stretch the fibres in this suit. Sign up for a free introductory class at a local studio, or learn the simple 10-minute Sun Salutation series outlined on page 24.

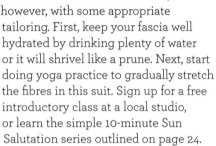

Roll it away

Try this simple experiment for one week. Each day while you're sitting at your desk or on the sofa, slowly roll your head and neck three times clockwise and three times anticlockwise. At first you'll hear lots of crackling, which is normal, but by the end of the week, these noises will mostly disappear. Regular yoga practice quiets and loosens your entire body in the same way. Find similar soothing moves for the joints that are bothering you most, and do them each day.

Live low-impact

Just like a car's suspension, your fascial system gets creaky over time. The vibrations from all the roads we travel and the potholes we hit take their toll. So minimise the damage by avoiding repetitive high-impact activities like running or jumping on hard surfaces. Stay aerobically fit with low-impact sports, such as walking, swimming and cycling.

Tuna out the pain

While research on glucosamine, chondroitin, SAM-e, vitamin E and other natural joint-pain relievers remains inconclusive, there is one supplement that appears to be effective. Studies show that omega-3 fatty acids (fish oil) reduce inflammation in joints and throughout the body, which benefits the heart. Salmon, mackerel and tuna are great natural sources.

Reevaluate cholesterol medication

Joint pain is a common side effect of some cholesterol-lowering drugs. So if your aches arrived with your new prescription, see your doctor.

MATTRESS MATTERS If your current mattress was bought in the 20th century, it could be the reason why you're feeling so battle weary. Sleep expert James B. Maas recommends buying a new one at least every decade. Forgotten how old yours is? 'If you've recently had a better night's sleep in a hotel or even a tent, it is probably shot,' he says. 'Find a new one that keeps your head, neck and spine aligned as if you were standing.' Oh, and write an expiration date of 10 years in the future on the tag so you'll know when to replace it.

End **knee pain** pronto

If your knees ache so much that even getting down on them to pray for help is out of the question, here are some potentially heaven-sent solutions.

Get a 4-for-1 deal

For every pound of weight you lose, the stress on your knees drops fourfold. For example, losing 5kg lightens their load by the equivalent of 20 kg, 10 by 40, 15 by 60 and so on. Weight loss is the simplest, most effective thing you can do to pull your joints back from their aching point.

Examine your sole

Look at the bottoms of your favourite shoes. If they're worn consistently along the outsides (or insides), then the natural roll of your feet while you walk or run may be twisting your knees. A podiatrist, or foot doctor, can design shoe inserts called orthotics to balance things out. Shoes themselves can also cause knee trouble. On days when you ache, note which ones you were wearing. Sometimes alleviating the pain is as simple as (yes!) going shopping for new ones.

Do some quad pumps

If you spend most of the day seated and it's a dull knee ache that's plaguing you, your joints may not be getting enough lubrication (such as blood, oxygen and nutrients). While seated, extend your legs with heels on the floor, contract both thigh muscles for a few seconds, then release and repeat 11 more times. Get into the habit of also doing this exercise during meetings, bus journeys, flights and long dinners.

Make this a mealtime standard

Studies show that three of the best foods for your knees are soy, fish and fruit. The first two supply anti-inflammatory

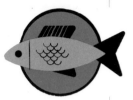

compounds, while the last provides vitamin C, all of which nourish the knee. Try combining the trio in a meal. Have salmon topped with kiwi/orange/mango salsa and a glass of soy milk. Or head to your nearest Japanese restaurant and order mackerel, tuna and salmon sashimi with edamame (soy beans) on the side.

Exercise more softly

You don't have to beat your body up to get a good workout. Brisk walking, swimming and cycling are low-impact activities that are kind to knees. If you're cycling, just remember to have your bike professionally fitted at a bike shop and, whenever you're exercising outdoors, cover your knees when temperatures dip below 16°C (60°F).

Recipe for relief

For those days when you overdo it (and get a headache to boot), follow this easy recipe for scoring some relief:

1. *Ingredients/Supplies*

   ▸▸ 350ml water

   ▸▸ 120ml surgical spirit

   ▸▸ 1 zip-seal plastic freezer bag (litre size)

2. *Pour water and alcohol into bag, seal and freeze. The alcohol in the surgical spirit will keep the water from completely freezing, leaving you with a mouldable slush that conforms perfectly to knees (and foreheads).*

3. *Lean back, say Ahhh.*

Prevent Alzheimer's

There's a retired man in our neighbourhood who we've known for years. On summer evenings he'd sit on his porch listening to the football. But the last time we stopped to chat, he didn't know the score or even who we were. His wife told us he'd been diagnosed with Alzheimer's. This debilitating disease is now a leading cause of death in the UK and the only one in the top 10 that cannot be slowed or cured. But that doesn't mean we're defenceless. Here's the best stay-sharp plan we know.

Don't waste money on brain boosters
Lots of vitamins and supplements claim to enhance brain health, but don't swallow that hype. Products that contain a variety of brain-boosting herbs and even those that deliver just one, like ginkgo biloba, have little if any supporting research, says brain expert Thomas Crook III, PhD.

Strengthen the heart; protect the brain
The brain is a highly vascular organ, meaning it's full of blood vessels. When you're concentrating, it can use up to 50 per cent of the body's total available fuel and oxygen. That means anything that's beneficial for the heart and circulatory system is also good for the brain. Exercising, eating less saturated fat and more fruits and vegetables, not smoking, controlling cholesterol… the prescription isn't any different. In fact, Alzheimer's may be a side effect of heart disease.

Befriend your local fishmonger
Eating three servings of fish per week may lower your risk of Alzheimer's by 50 per cent. Scientists believe this is due to specific compounds called omega-3 fatty acids. These bolster the cardiovascular system and promote brain growth and development. (One of these compounds, DHA, is actually

abundant in mother's milk.) The latest thinking, however, is that omega-3s are best utilised by the body when ingested naturally rather than as supplements.

Be a lifelong learner

Whether you're studying a second language, researching a topic on the internet, or just doing the Sunday crossword, the effort involved is mental exercise. Learning is Zumba for the brain.

Think about what you drink

To keep your brain functioning at a high level, drink plenty of water. However, there's no proven benefit to special concoctions such as SmartWater. There is some evidence that caffeine, in moderation, may be protective of memory. And when it comes to alcohol, one large study found that those who downed more than 14 drinks per week suffered a 1.6 per cent reduction in relative brain volume.

Sleep eight to nine hours nightly

Your brain is still on while your body is off. It's operating at a maintenance and restorative level that's essential to long-term function and health. Being well rested is not just a way to be productive the next day but also well into the future.

A BRAIN ON TOP OF ITS GAME

20 to 25 per cent ▸▸ The amount of total blood volume delivered to the brain with every heartbeat

100 billion ▸▸ The number of nerve cells or neurons in an adult brain

100 trillion ▸▸ The number of connection points or synapses between those cells (the so-called neuron forest)

Put a stop to
cold sores

Although they're medically insignificant, these little devils can cause a great deal of personal hell because they're so visible and unsightly. And because cold sores often are sparked by stress, they always seem to appear at the worst possible times (important presentations, meetings, holidays, dates). Unfortunately, there's no cure for the herpes simplex viruses that cause these bothersome blisters, but their frequency and duration can be managed quite well. Assuming you're already carrying the virus (as around 70 per cent of adult British people are), here's how to be a more successful sore loser.

Avoid pulling the typical triggers
The virus that causes cold sores lies dormant until something awakens it. These triggers include prolonged sun exposure (without using a lip balm of SPF 15 or higher), lack of sleep, anxiety, colds and flu, and any sort of lip trauma (so go easy on the kissing, lover). There is also some evidence that arginine, an amino acid found in shellfish, spinach, sesame seeds, turkey and many other foods causes them. To see if you're sensitive, review your diet in the days before an outbreak.

Put it on ice
As soon as you feel a lip tingle or itch, wrap an ice cube in a thin towel and hold it on the spot for a few minutes. Do this repeatedly for one and a half to two hours and the sore may either never blossom or be less severe.

Find your best defence

There are lots of home remedies with some supporting research that may or may not work for you. When an outbreak seems imminent or is in progress, try taking aspirin (125mg daily), lysine (1,000 to 3,000mg daily), echinacea (1,200mg daily), quercetin (1,000mg daily) or applying lemon balm ointment. Don't do everything at once; use a process of elimination.

Arm yourself with antivirals

If you don't want to waste time experimenting with home remedies, ask your doctor about oral and topical prescription medications that can minimise outbreaks and their severity. These include valacyclovir (Valtrex), famciclovir (Famvir) and acyclovir (Zovirax). A cream with some positive supporting research in the US is docosanol (Abreva), which is available online.

Wait it out

The frequency of outbreaks tends to decrease with age, so if you can use the previous strategies to keep them at bay, by age 35 or so they should become less of a worry.

KEEP YOUR SISTER-IN-LAW AWAY

Q: Most people acquire oral herpes as children. How do they get it?

A: A kiss from a friend or relative, whether they're symptomatic at the time or not.

Never suffer
from osteoporosis

By the time you're 18 (for women) or 20 (for men), you have 85 to 90 per cent of the bone mass you'll have for life. Your job then becomes one of maintenance. If you're not careful, you can lose 0.6 to 1.0 per cent of your bone density every year, which in time can leave your skeleton so brittle that sneezing could cause a fracture. Although osteoporosis has traditionally been regarded as a postmenopausal women's disease, 20 per cent of sufferers are men. But relax. If you're smart, there's no need to ever get bent out of shape.

Bone up on family history

Osteoporosis has a large genetic component. Look for telltale signs of osteoporosis (height loss, forward-curving spine) in your parents and grandparents. You may be offered a DXA scan, a type of X-ray that measures bone mineral density (BMD), if you are considered at high risk of having or developing osteoporosis.

Calculate your calcium

Bone is living tissue, and calcium is the mineral that sustains it. Adults need 1,000 mg (under age 50) to 1,200mg (over age 50) daily. Ideally, this should come from a mix of natural sources such as dairy, broccoli, beans, tofu and dark, leafy greens. (A recent study in the *British Medical Journal* suggests calcium supplements raise the risk of heart attacks.) Periodic blood and urine tests can be done to monitor levels.

Mobilise your D-fence

Calcium may be the major construction material in bone, but vitamin D is the foreman that makes sure it's being efficiently used. Adults need 400 to 800 IU (under age 50) and 800 to

1,000 IU (over age 50) daily. The easiest way to get your dose is by spending 10 to 15 minutes outdoors each day before applying sunscreen.

Exercise smarter

There are two types of exercise that benefit bone most. The first is weight-bearing activity, like walking and tennis, which utilises the skeleton for support and impact-resistance. (Non-weight-bearing activities, like swimming and cycling, do not.) The second type is resistance training, which for most people means lifting weights. In fact, bone responds just like muscle does to weight lifting, becoming bigger, denser and stronger.

Be wary of these

According to the National Osteoporosis Society, ingesting too much protein and sodium may promote calcium and bone loss. Studies point to high-protein fad diets and fizzy drinks in particular.

BUILD BETTER BALANCE WITH ONE MOVE There's an important component of fitness beyond strength, endurance and flexibility that most people neglect. It's balance, and it becomes increasingly vital with age. The evidence? A shocking 24 per cent of hip-fracture patients over 50 die in the year following their fracture. Whether you have osteoporosis or not, preventing a fall is a smart health move. Hone it by making this simple exercise a regular part of your workout:

Stand with a wall or other sturdy object on your left, pick a stationary focal point directly ahead, and slowly raise your right leg until the knee is bent at 90 degrees and your thigh is parallel to the floor. With your hands at your sides, maintain your gaze and take five full breaths. Lower that leg, turn around (wall on your right now) and repeat with the left leg. Once this becomes easy, try straightening the raised leg and pointing the toe while lifting it as high as possible.

Best 40+-minute workout:
Strength training

Whenever you have more time to exercise, the best way to spend it is by strength training. Regardless of age, it will tone and build muscle. And since muscle tissue requires more energy to sustain than fat tissue, you'll burn calories even while at rest and lose weight faster. Resistance training also increases bone density, which fights osteoporosis, as well as just helping us cope with the physical demands of life. Plus, when done in a circuit with little rest in between exercises, it becomes aerobic.

What follows is a total-body strength workout that uses dumbbells for most exercises and takes 40 minutes or more to complete. Start by doing one set of 8 to 12 repetitions for each exercise at a comfortable pace and with a manageable weight. Once that becomes easy, add more weight, a second or third set of reps, or rest less in between exercises.

Warm up

Do 5 minutes of activity that gets your blood flowing and your muscles moving. Great choices include walking in place, lifting your knees high as you go; walking on a treadmill; peddling on a stationary bike; going up and down stairs; or doing 25 to 50 jumping jacks.

Lunge

- *quadriceps*
- *hamstrings*
- *buttocks*

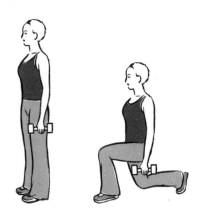

Stand tall with feet hip-width apart and dumbbells at your sides. Take a big step forwards with your left foot, keeping your upper body perpendicular to the ground and left knee over the ankle. You'll end up on the ball of your right foot with that knee bent. Hold the lunge for a few seconds, then step back to the start position and repeat with the opposite leg. That's one rep.

Calf raise

- *calves*

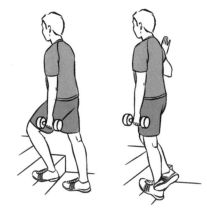

While holding a dumbbell in your left hand at your side, put the toes of your left foot on a bottom stair. Next, while resting your opposite hand on the wall or banister for stability, tuck your right foot behind your left ankle and slowly rise up and down on your toes. Do one set, then switch legs.

Bent-over row

- *lower back*
- *shoulders*

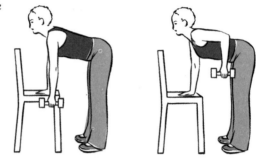

With a dumbbell in your left hand, bend over and rest your right hand on a chair seat. Ground yourself, then pull the weight up towards your underarm while keeping that elbow close to your side. Slowly lower it. That's one rep. After completing your reps on this side, move the weight to the other hand and repeat.

Upright row

- *forearms*
- *shoulders*
- *upper back*

Stand tall with feet hip-width apart and a dumbbell in each hand, palms facing the front of your thighs. Line the weights up along the front of your body until your elbows are parallel to the floor. Pause and return to the start position. That's one rep.

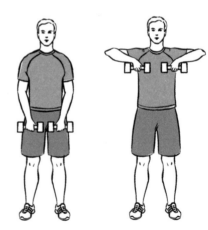

Finding solutions

Push-up

- *chest*
- *arms*

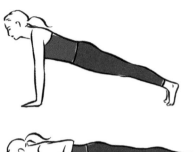

Start in a plank position with hands directly beneath shoulders. While keeping your elbows tucked, slowly lower yourself to the floor and then press back up. If this is too difficult, put your knees on the ground.

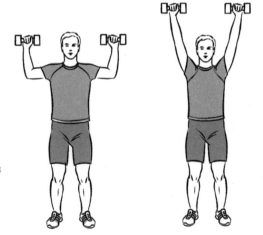

Push press

- *shoulders*
- *arms*

Stand tall with feet hip-width apart while holding a dumbbell in each hand. Raise both arms until the elbows are bent 90 degrees, with palms facing forwards and knees bent. Now press both weights overhead as you straighten your legs. Then lower the dumbbells back to the bent elbows position as you squat again. That's one rep.

Opposite arm/opposite leg

- *lower back*
- *posterior legs*
- *shoulders*

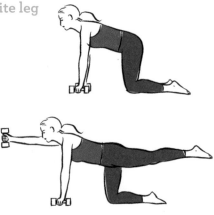

Assume a table position on the floor, with knees directly under hips and each hand grasping a dumbbell (directly under shoulders, palms turned in). Raise and extend your left leg while doing the same with your right arm. Pause for 2 or 3 seconds with that leg and arm parallel to the ground, then lower and repeat on the other side. That's one rep.

Crunch

- *abdominals*

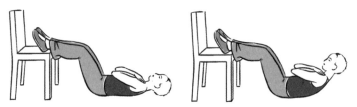

Lie on your back with knees bent and feet on a chair seat. Fold your arms across your chest with fingertips touching opposite shoulders. While keeping your elbows and chin tucked in, slowly curl your upper body towards your legs, hold for a few seconds and then slowly lower down.

Cool down
5 minutes (light stretching)

PERSONAL N●TES

{ How do I waste time, and how can I **better** use that **time?** }

Cut your
cholesterol, naturally

Cholesterol-lowering drugs are cheap and effective. So why not just pop a daily pill and stop worrying about clogged arteries? If your doctor says you need them, we have no argument. But if it's partly your decision, consider:

▶▶ *Too many people nowadays address every problem with a pill until their medicine cabinet looks like a Boots shelf. Overmedication is a serious health problem in itself.*

▶▶ *Not addressing the root causes of high cholesterol, such as a poor diet and/or a sedentary lifestyle puts you at risk of developing other chronic illnesses, such as hypertension and diabetes.*

So while swallowing a pill may seem like the simplest solution, you might be making it harder on yourself in the long term. Make sense? Good. Now let's begin with the three most effective strategies for managing cholesterol naturally.

Rough up your diet

The number-one foodstuff for lowering cholesterol, according to doctors at the Mayo Clinic in the US, is soluble fibre. It reduces the absorption of cholesterol into the blood while targeting its worst component (LDL). There are an overwhelming array of cholesterol-fighting foods and claims, but people with diets highest in fibre reduce their risk of heart disease by nearly a third. The recommended daily allowance is 24 grams. Meeting that requirement will mean eating more fruits and vegetables, less junk food and fewer calories overall (because fibre-rich foods fill you up). More fibre also means less saturated fat, which Heart UK, Britain's cholesterol charity, says should amount to less than 10 per cent of your daily diet. Porridge, kidney beans, apples, pears, barley and apricots are all soluble superstars.

Follow this training plan

Although any exercise provides heart and health benefits, there are particular ones that seem to control cholesterol best. The more you work out aerobically, as measured by duration or distance, the better the results. (Intensity doesn't matter as much.) Research also shows that strength training is effective for improving cholesterol profiles (lowers LDL while raising HDL). So combine the two in a weekly programme that alternates three days of longer walks, runs or bike rides at a moderate pace with three days of total-body resistance training. (If you've been sedentary, work up to these levels slowly under the guidance of a doctor and trainer.)

Become less of a man (or woman)

Losing weight – even as little as 4 or 5kg – produces beneficial changes in cholesterol. Even better news: if you follow our first two tips, you won't have to do anything extra to achieve this. You'll drop weight automatically.

POP, POP, POP...

17.8 ‣ Average number of prescription items dispensed by the NHS in 2010 per head of population (up from 11.2 in 2000)

50 ‣ Per cent of over 65s taking five or more drugs

£8.8 billion ‣ Total NHS prescription drugs bill for England in 2011

3 ‣ Rank of cholesterol-lowering medicines among all drugs prescribed by the NHS

61.5 million ‣ Number of prescriptions written in 2011 for cholesterol-lowering drugs

7 million ‣ Estimated number of people taking statins in the UK

Soothe a
sore muscle

We know, we know. You're constantly being told to exercise more. But when you finally follow through, you feel worse than before. Muscle soreness can leave you hobbling for days. Truth is, if you're aching that much, you overdid it. When you exercise again, do a little less and progress gradually from week to week. Meanwhile, you need relief. Here's how to provide it.

Be proud of yourself
If you exercised yesterday and your muscles are mildly sore today, that means you had a productive workout. Muscles require a small degree of damage in order to grow and develop. 'If you jog the same two miles at the same pace day after day, you will never become faster or stronger,' explains Dr. Gabe Mirkin. 'All improvement in any muscle function comes from stressing and recovering.'

Lactic acid has nothing to do with it
Experts used to think that this caustic substance built up in the muscle during exercise and caused the resulting soreness. But that's not the case, says Dr. Mirkin, who is certified by the American Board of Sports Medicine. It's actually damage to the muscle fibres themselves that's the source of the ache. Biopsies reveal actual bleeding in the muscle tissue.

Pass up the painkillers
Most people reach immediately for ibuprofen and other nonsteroidal anti-inflammatories (NSAIDs) when muscle soreness strikes. But there's conflicting evidence as to how helpful these are after exercise. So unless the ache is severe, it might be better to just tough it out.

Ice the inflammation

To help soothe the soreness, cut 3-cm slits in a few tennis balls, fill them about 75 per cent with water, and freeze. They're great for rolling over muscles to reduce inflammation, plus their furry surface prevents skin irritation.

Pop some polyphenols

These are antioxidants from plant foods that work in the body to enhance health. They are prevalent in fruits, vegetables, whole grains and legumes, and have recently been found to reduce muscle inflammation and its resulting tenderness. In fact, they appear to work better than NSAIDs. Refining of foods removes polyphenols, so eat fresh or freshly cooked foods.

Take it easy for the next few days

Depending on how tender your muscles feel, either rest entirely or exercise lightly. All aches should be gone before working out hard again. Incidentally, Dr Mirkin says stretching muscles after exercise won't prevent soreness because contracted muscle fibres are not to blame.

GET RID OF A SIDE STITCH These sharp pains are caused by a spasm in the diaphragm muscle or its surrounding tissue. To prevent it, avoid eating a couple hours prior to exercising. If one hits, try one or both of these remedies to get relief quick:

▸▸ **Give yourself the fingers:** press two fingers up and in towards the hurt just below the ribs and take deep breaths. This should relax the spasm.

▸▸ **Stretch that side:** stand and raise your right arm overhead (if the stitch is on the right side) and bend to the left. If the stitch is on the opposite side, do the reverse.

Lower your cancer risk

We're not going to dwell on the obvious. Avoiding tobacco, losing weight, exercising regularly, wearing sunscreen, having recommended tests and eating lots of whole foods are all proven cancer fighters. This, you should already know. Here are some highly effective strategies based on the latest research that you may underestimate or not be aware of at all.

Update your family history
Your doctor will always ask if there have been any changes in your health since your last visit. Answer this question *broadly,* letting him know if any immediate family members have recently been diagnosed with a disease. Knowing if a relative has breast or colon cancer, for instance, will help him better gauge your risk and may affect the screenings he recommends.

Keep a check on sunscreens
Sunscreen testing and labelling started to change from 2008 following a European Commission recommendation aimed at keeping sun safety simple. Over the coming years we'll be seeing fewer SPF numbers to help simplify choice, and an indication of the type of protection that product gives you (low to very high). Cancer Research UK and the Department of Health recommend an SPF of at least 15, with a star rating of four stars or more to protect against UVA. Stay up to date at sunsmart.org.uk.

Consider the wonder drug
In a study tracking more than 25,000 patients, those taking a daily low-dose aspirin had a 21 per cent lower risk of dying from cancer than those who didn't swallow one. More specifically, rates of lung cancer in the group dropped 30 per cent, colorectal cancer 40 per cent and oesophageal cancer 60 per

cent. Consult with your doctor first, however, since aspirin can cause stomach bleeding and other problems.

Trim your body fat

Britain has the third-highest rate of increase in obesity in the world, with levels rapidly approaching those in the US. According to Cancer Research UK, obesity is responsible for about 7 per cent of the UK's cancer deaths. Post-menopausal women who are overweight run twice the risk of getting breast cancer and studies pointed to expanding waistlines as being the best indicator of future incidence of colon cancers. Body fat promotes cancer by raising oestrogen levels, interfering with insulin production and causing chronic inflammation.

Cut back on the booze

Alcohol is now known to be responsible for seven types of cancer. And, unfortunately, as little as three units a day can increase your risk of bowel, breast, mouth, food pipe and throat cancers. The risk increases the more you drink. Make sure you stick to one small drink a day (about two units) for women or two (three to four units) for men.

Bookmark this site

If you have a family history of cancer or if avoiding it is a health priority, the website of Cancer Research UK (cancerresearchuk.org) is an indispensable resource. In researching this book, we visited hundreds of health sites, and it is among the most comprehensive, authoritative and helpful. Its Cancer Help patient information microsite is truly comprehensive and its news section is particularly good for summarising the latest studies in layman's terms.

Don't be blind to
sight problems

We worry that a heart attack or arthritis will compromise our retirement years, but one-third of us will have our independence severely curtailed by something we rarely even consider. Vision loss or blindness from cataracts, diabetic retinopathy, glaucoma and macular degeneration is forecast to rise 50 per cent by 2020. This is partially due to people living longer, but also to many of us just taking our eyesight for granted. Not any more.

Follow a check-up schedule
Most vision problems can be managed or corrected if diagnosed early. In your 40s, 50s and early 60s, you should have a complete eye examination every two to four years. After age 65 it should be annual. Senior citizens (60 and over) are entitled to free eye tests.

Avoid or reverse diabetes
People with diabetes (Types 1 and 2) are 25 times more likely to lose their vision than people without the disease. See page 118 for our best tips on preventing diabetes. Or if you've already been diagnosed, consider this an additional incentive to manage it more stringently.

Go Hollywood
The sun's UV rays can fry your eyes just as they can your skin. To avoid corneal sunburn, wear wraparound-style sunglasses that block 100 per cent of all UV light. You can also get UV coatings on contact lenses.

Eat more kale than carrots

Your mum was half right: carrots do contain lots of eye-nourishing nutrients. But the best food for your vision is dark green leafy vegetables, like spinach, Swiss chard and especially kale. They contain lutein and zeaxanthin, antioxidants that may even reduce the progression of age-related macular degeneration. If you're not a fan of their taste, toss a handful into stir-fries, soups and pasta sauces, where you'll barely notice them. Overall, the more fruits, vegetables and whole foods in your diet, the healthier your eyes will be.

Wear eye protection

Most eye injuries don't occur on assembly lines or sports fields. They happen doing everyday household DIY and chores. Buy a few pairs of European Standard-approved safety goggles and put a set in the garage, basement, kitchen, shed and wherever else they'll be handy.

See into the future

To actually experience what it's like to have cataracts, diabetic retinopathy, glaucoma or macular degeneration, visit eyecareamerica.org and click on 'eye disease simulators'. If this doesn't prompt you to take better care of your peepers, nothing will.

DO YOU HAVE MACULAR DEGENERATION? Go to macular.org/chart.html for a test. It is called Amsler's Grid. To use it, hold a printout of the page at arm's length and eye level (with reading glasses on, if necessary). Cover one eye and gaze at the centre dot, then repeat with the opposite eye. If any lines are distorted or missing, see an eye specialist for further testing.

Let your pet
be your doctor

One day in the not-too distant future, you may encounter sniffer dogs in Outpatients, just like you do at the airport. Researchers are finding that certain breeds of dog can detect cancers (prostate, colon, skin, lung, bowel, breast), sense impending hypoglycemic episodes and may even be able to warn of seizures (see 'Good Boy' on page 125). Although exactly how they do this is unclear, it's believed they can pick out a disease's odour, as well as subtle behavioural changes in people. But you don't have to wait until pooch prevention is perfected. There are other ways you can use a pet to make yourself and your family healthier.

Fitness partner
One of the best ways to get fit and stay fit is to recruit an exercise buddy – someone who'll goad you into working out when you don't feel like it. Well, that partner doesn't have to be human. An active dog that shows up each morning with leash in mouth is just as difficult to let down.

Stress reducer
Simply petting an animal lowers blood pressure and decreases heart rate. In a classic study of stockbrokers with hypertension, those who took in a dog or cat were better able to handle job pressure.

Heart builder
Dog owners generally have lower levels of triglercerides and male pet owners have lower LDL (bad) cholesterol levels, meaning they have less risk of heart disease. On a broader level, caring for a pet and seeing an appreciative tail wag encourages feelings of well-being that make people feel happier, better

connected and perhaps most importantly, unconditionally loved. Certain groups of patients (the elderly, children and the terminally ill) have been shown to benefit from contact with specially trained animals.

Habit breaker

Let's say you want your dog's help to quit smoking. First, use a treat to teach your pet to bark on command when ordering, 'Speak!' Once he's mastered this, hold up a pack of cigarettes, give the same command, and then reward him when he cooperates. In no time he'll be barking whenever you reach for your ciggies, which will hopefully serve as a reminder not to light up. The same strategy can be creatively applied to any bad habit you're trying to kick, such as biting nails or wolfing down snacks.

Allergy fighter

Contrary to popular belief, having a furry pet in the house appears to help immunise some kids to allergens and boost their immune systems. However, if your youngster is seriously allergic, buy the cutest, most cuddly stuffed animal you can find. A couple of studies have found that these help children better cope with stress. While you're at it, buy one for yourself. No one has to know.

BUT DON'T LET HIM DO THIS Mattress-manufacturer Sealy found that 67 per cent of pet owners regularly sleep with their dogs and cats. Thirty-eight per cent, however, confessed that their animals were far from perfect sleepers and disturbed their night's rest. US researchers at the Mayo Clinic Sleep Disorders Centre found that snoring, especially among dogs, was a common culprit.

Boost your **fertility**

You might have worried about it happening all through your wanton youth. But now that you're actually trying to have a baby and it's not happening, you're even more anxious. You're not alone. Approximately 3.5 million people in the UK have difficulty conceiving, and it can be emotionally as well as financially draining. But there are some simple lifestyle changes that can make a big difference. Try these before seeing a specialist.

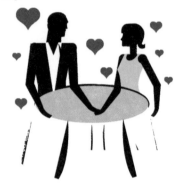

Calculate your baby-making index

You've probably heard of BMI (body mass index) as a gauge for whether you're under- or overweight. But it can also be viewed as the baby-making index because body fat plays a critical role in reproduction. Go to bhf.org.uk/bmi/BMI_Calc.html and calculate BMI for you and your partner. If one or both of you are below or above the norm, your fertility is being compromised. If you're having problems conceiving, address any weight issues first.

Clear the air

Women who smoke have a 60 per cent greater risk of infertility than those who don't. And although smoking's effect on the male reproductive system doesn't appear to be as dramatic, if a spouse puffs, secondhand smoke is nearly as destructive. Fortunately, quitting has immediate benefits, with fertility usually returning to normal within a year.

Don't go to extremes
Whether it's alcohol, caffeine or even exercise, your new mantra should be moderation. Consuming more than two alcoholic drinks or more than five cups of coffee (totalling 500mg of caffeine) daily has been shown to decrease fertility in women. Likewise, exercising for more than an hour per day can interfere with ovulation.

Brush and floss your teeth daily
Women who are trying to get pregnant should make sure they look after their dental hygiene. A Swedish study suggests gum disease can lengthen the time it takes for a woman to become pregnant. Those who flossed regularly reduced the time it took to get pregnant by 30 per cent. This may be because of the low-grade inflammation created by infected gums.

Scrutinise that scrotum
A common cause of male infertility is varicoceles – dilated or varicose veins in the scrotum. Forty per cent of men experiencing infertility have them. After a warm shower, when things are most relaxed, check for what will feel like a small ball of worms or even spaghetti in either sack. A doctor should check anything suspicious.

Make love more often
Many couples believe that frequent ejaculation decreases sperm count. Not so. Reproductive efficiency, as those romantic researchers like to call it, is highest when intercourse occurs every one to two days. Incidentally, no one sexual position is better (or worse) for conception than another, but of course, you're free to continue the research.

Relax
That's right. Resign yourself to a kidless life if that's what it takes to notch down the pressure. Stress plays havoc with fertility, too.

A TRUE ROMANTIC MEAL Although research is continuing, there appear to be certain foods that boost fertility. So we've combined them into one meal. Don't forget the candles.

Appetiser
▸▸ **Oysters:** Zinc promotes semen production and ovulation.

Entrée
▸▸ **Salmon:** Omega-3 fatty acids increase blood flow to the uterus.

▸▸ **Steamed broccoli:** Foods high in vitamin C increase fertility.

▸▸ **Lentils:** Beans have folate, which increases sperm count and density.

▸▸ **Wine:** Time to conceive for women who have an occasional glass is shorter than for teetotalers, according to a Danish study.

Dessert
▸▸ **Ice cream:** A twice-weekly 120ml serving of full-fat dairy increased the odds of pregnancy in a study of 19,000 nurses.

PERSONAL N●TES

{ What can I do to make my **relationship** healthier for me? }

Soothe a sore throat

Sore throats are worrying because their cause is often unclear. Is it a sign of impeding cold or flu, or is it the result of yet another night of karaoke you hope didn't make it on to YouTube? Or maybe it's something worse – like a strep infection, glandular fever or even the throat cancer that actor Michael Douglas had. Before you stress out, here's some diagnostic advice that's easy to swallow.

Open wide and take a photo

To get a rough idea of what's going on in there, snap a shot of the back of your throat. At the very least, it'll make an interesting addition to your Facebook page. And if things look angry and inflamed, you'll have confirmed an infection.

Wait out a virus

The same viruses that trigger colds and flu cause most sore throats. So if you also have the sniffles and your throat is just mildly sore, the best treatment is to gargle, sip liquids, suck lozenges and let the bug run its course (usually five to seven days). *Don't* take antibiotics; they do nothing for viral infections. (Note: if these symptoms persist and are accompanied by swollen lymph nodes in the neck and armpits, plus fatigue and a high temperature, see a doctor as it could be glandular fever.)

Test for bacteria

If your sore throat is severe with a high fever and swollen glands or lasts beyond a week, the infection could be bacterial. This is more serious and needs a doctor's attention. The good news is that bacterial infections do respond to antibiotics.

Don't mess around with recurrent ones

If you're regularly plagued by a sore throat, it could be tonsillitis or, if the symptoms are seasonal, allergy related. Even worse, if a sore throat keeps returning, get checked for throat cancer. There's one type – oropharyngeal cancer – that affects both smokers and nonsmokers and is linked to the same virus (HPV) that's linked to cervical cancer. It's on the rise.

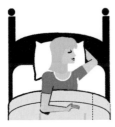

Revamp your bedroom

When there are no visible signs of inflammation or other symptoms but your throat is scratchy in the morning, it could be a simple case of sleeping with your mouth open or inhaling dry air. Try raising your head above your stomach with a more supportive pillow or by putting bricks under the two top bed legs. If that doesn't work, put a humidifier in the room.

A GAGGLE OF GARGLES Gargling is one of the oldest and most effective home remedies for soothing a sore throat. Experiment with these to find the one that works best for you:

▶▶ **The Classic:** 225ml warm water with ¼ teaspoon salt.

▶▶ **The Classic Plus:** Same as above but with an additional tablespoon of Listerine (for germ killing).

▶▶ **The New Favourite:** 225ml warm water with 1 teaspoon lemon juice. (The astringent juice shrinks swollen tissue, while the acid fights viruses and bacteria.)

▶▶ **The No Hassle:** Buy a ready-made mouthwash at the chemist, such as 'Difflam Oral Rinse'. Use undiluted every one and a half to three hours for no more than seven days.

▶▶ **The Nightcap:** 120ml warm water, juice from ½ lemon, 1 teaspoon powdered ginger, 1 teaspoon honey. (Coats the throat and has mild antibacterial properties.)

Make these health moves in
your
60s (and beyond)

What	When
Routine checks/exams	
Complete health check-up	Every 5 years
Blood pressure	Every 5 years *(more frequently if at risk; ask your doctor)*
Cholesterol	Every 5 years *(more frequently if at risk; ask your doctor)*
Blood glucose	Every 5 years *(annually if you're overweight or have a family history of Type 1 diabetes)*
Eyesight	Annually
Teeth	At least every 2 years *(seek guidance from your dentist)*
Body mass index (BMI)	Every 6 months
Prostate specific antigen (PSA)	Once *(discuss with your doctor)*
Faecal occult blood	Every 2 years
Bone density	Only if at risk *(alert your doctor if you have a family history of osteoporosis)*
Mammogram	Every 3 years
Cervical smear test	Every 5 years < 64
Abdominal aortic aneurysm	One ultrasound scan for men at age 65

ome very smart people spend their entire lives saving for their retirement years, only to find that when the time arrives, health is the new wealth. Hopefully, your personal portfolio is robust with this investment and your interest is compounding. But even if it isn't, there's still plenty of time to catch up. Remember: age alone doesn't cause you to become sick or feeble. Decline is a function of how you choose to live.

Innoculations

Influenza	Annually *(free on the NHS to over 65s)*
Pneumonia	Once per lifetime *(available on the NHS to over 65s)*
Others	If missed in prior decades *(see page 42)*

General

Volunteer.	Giving back lowers risk of death.
Make more friends.	Social support boosts immunity.
Lift weights/eat protein.	Fights muscle/strength loss.
Go back to school.	Learning promotes brain growth.

Make these health moves in your 60s (and beyond)

Find allergy relief

First, look on the bright side. If your allergies to pollen, dust, mould, pet dander or whatever else are making you miserable, it could mean you have a lower risk of brain tumours and cancer. Scientists theorise that since allergies are caused by an overactive immune system, such a SWAT-like response could ward off other cellular invaders as well. So when the sniffles strike, keep that in mind. In the meantime...

Hit the bedroom hard

Since you spend about a third of your life sleeping, direct most of your home allergy-proofing efforts here. Besides regular cleaning, get rid of carpeting and heavy curtains that can harbour allergens, keep windows and doors closed (especially to a damp bathroom) and move Fluffy out. (We're talking about your pet, not your spouse.) Also, seal pillows and mattresses inside allergen-impermeable covers. And if you can't launder all the bedding weekly (in 60°C water as recommended), at least wash the pillowcases, since your face presses against them all night.

Take better care of your hair

Your hairdo is out in the world all day collecting who knows what, so don't go to bed without washing it. (Or bring back the nightcap – nonalcoholic.) Similarly, one study found that men who scrubbed their moustache twice daily with liquid soap needed fewer antihistamines and decongestants.

Check the probability of nose precipitation

You plan your activities around the weather, so why not pay similar attention to the allergy forecast? You'll find pollen counts on most weather websites, including that of the Met Office (metoffice.gov.uk/health/public/pollen-forecast). On days when things look threatening, limit outdoor activities and keep all windows closed.

Try one of these

Claritin was the most recommended over-the-counter antihistamine by pharmacists in a recent survey, and its generic form (loratadine) was named a 'best buy' by *Consumer Reports Health*. It causes less drowsiness than traditional antihistamines, and only one dose is needed every 12 or 24 hours. Antihistamines work best, though, when taken *before* allergy symptoms hit.

Rinse your nasal passages daily

Just as a rain shower rinses pollen from the air, a saline rinse washes allergens from your nasal passages. To make your own saline rinse, mix ½ teaspoon salt, ½ teaspoon bicarbonate of soda and 500ml (1 pint) warm tap water. To get it into your nose, use an infant ear bulb-syringe or a neti pot (a small container with a spout), available from health food shops and pharmacies. Lean over a sink and turn your head so that your left nostril points downwards. Gently flush your right nostril with 250ml (5 teaspoons) of saline, which will drain out through your left nostril. When you're finished, gently blow your nose. Repeat with the other nostril.

IT COULD BE WORSE: 5 REALLY WEIRD ALLERGIES

▸▸ **Kissing:** Some people with food allergies can have a reaction after smooching someone who ate what they're sensitive to.

▸▸ **Sex:** It's possible to be allergic to spermicides, lubricants, latex and even semen.

▸▸ **Talking on the phone:** This allergy stems from prolonged exposure to the nickel inside most mobile phones. It causes itching in the cheeks and jaw.

▸▸ **Tattoos:** The colour pigments can trigger a reaction.

▸▸ **Wine:** Newly discovered 'glycoproteins' appear to be the culprit.

End **back pain** forever

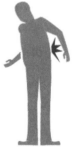

L ow back pain is the most common type of chronic pain, plaguing almost twice as many people as the next biggest hurt (headaches). Eighty per cent of adults will suffer a sore back at some point in life. Fortunately, most cases won't require hospitalisation or surgery and can be managed and even cured with lifestyle changes. Here are some little things you can do to make your spine smile.

Clean out your bag
One sneaky cause of chronic back pain is overloaded handbags, backpacks and briefcases. Hanging a heavy weight off one side of your body (when you're in heels, no less) stresses your entire skeleton as it tries to compensate. Weigh your bag on the bathroom scales. If it's more than 10 per cent of your body weight, pare it down (or buy a lighter one).

Carry less cash
Hey, big spender, sitting on a fat wallet all day twists the spine and compresses nerves in the buttocks and leg. Sciatica is the inflammation of those nerves. This problem is so common among men that it has a clinical name: wallet neuropathy.

Reach for heat before pills
When low back pain strikes, try treating it with ThermaCare HeatWraps rather than ibuprofen or acetaminophen. These wearable pads provide 40°C heat for up to eight hours. By increasing blood flow to the sore spot, they promote healing and mobility. Staying active is important because bed rest appears to make back pain worse if you have short-term (acute) back pain, but be careful and don't do anything that makes the pain worse.

Finding solutions

Get some trousers tailored

This is a quick and inexpensive way to determine if one of your legs is shorter than the other. Nobody's perfect, and any discrepancy greater than 1.5cm could affect your back. If the tailor detects a difference, put a Dr Scholl's–type lift in your shoe or consult a podiatrist about custom inserts.

Tune up your body mechanics

When standing for any length of time, get in the habit of keeping one foot in front of the other. When sitting at your desk or on a long flight, put something under your feet so your knees are slightly higher than your hips. Both ease pressure on the lower back.

Assume the position

The best sleeping position if you have a bad back is on your side with a pillow tucked between bent knees. Sleeping face up or down arches the spine and prevents it from fully relaxing. To keep from rolling onto your back or belly while you're unconscious, duct-tape a golf ball to the front and rear of your nightshirt. Chances are, you'll wake up feeling above par.

LET'S ROLL A recent study found the benefits of regular Swedish massage to be 'about as strong as medications, acupuncture, exercise and yoga' for treating back pain. But unless you're married to someone named Rolf or Inga, it may be an indulgence that's too expensive. Enter the high-density foam roller, a self-massage tool that's especially effective at working out kinks and promoting blood flow to the lower back. Simply roll around on top of it using your body weight for pressure. You can find foam rollers at most sports stores or online. It's an easy and cheap way to self-manage your own body.

Heal yourself
with mind power

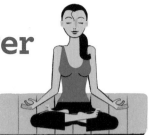

Although we tend to view body and mind as separate entities (thank you, all you Playboy bunnies), the two are intertwined in ways that medical science, despite all its progress, is just fathoming. But that needn't stop you from experimenting. Whether you're out to muster your defences for flu season or manage a chronic disease in yourself or a loved one, here's how to potentially recruit your greatest ally.

Learn the relaxation response

Harvard Medical School professor Herbert Benson, MD, estimates that 60 to 90 per cent of doctor visits are linked in some way to stress. So it follows that if you can learn to manage stress better, your health will automatically improve. The key, he says, is eliciting the 'relaxation response'. This is a deep but conscious state of rest that lowers metabolism, heart rate, respiration, blood pressure and muscle tension – all of which promotes healing and well-being. To learn it, sit quietly in a comfortable position, close your eyes and breathe slowly and naturally. Once you're relaxed, start repeating a personally meaningful word or phrase (such as love, peace, Hail Mary, John Lennon...). Continue for 10 to 20 minutes, practising twice daily. You should eventually feel more balanced.

Pop a placebo

You've no doubt heard about participants in clinical trials who were unknowingly given sugar pills yet experienced measurable positive effects. This is the power of belief at work. In fact, the American Cancer Society states that while placebos do not act on disease, 'they seem to have an effect in 1 out of 3 patients'. Although you can't evoke a placebo effect in yourself (because you know what's being done), if you're looking to ease the suffering of a chronically ill relative or friend, consider asking their doctor to 'prescribe' a placebo.

Say your prayers

There is some research supporting the long-held belief that praying, whether for yourself or others, can positively influence health. On one level, petitioning a Higher Power to intercede on your behalf counters feelings of stress and powerlessness. On another, being prayed for by others reinforces your connection with family and community, which can be empowering and actually speed healing. It doesn't even matter if the praying is done in church. A study of breast cancer patients who prayed in online support groups found evidence of lower negativity and higher well-being.

Be a little more optimistic

Having a positive outlook on life has been shown to lower the risk of heart disease and stroke, protect against breast cancer, and reduce the odds of dying from any cause compared to people who are more pessimistic. Isn't that terrific news?

MEDITATE WHILE YOU MOVE If sitting quietly trying to evoke the relaxation response drives you nuts, take a different approach: Do it while exercising. Instead of focusing on a word or phrase, let the movement be your mantra. For example, when walking outside or on a treadmill, bring your attention to each footfall – left/right/left/right. In other words, let its sound and feel be your metronome. This is what's known as 'mindful exercise'. After a while it can put you in a zone that is just as rejuvenating and nourishing as conventional meditation.

PROJECT STAFF
Writer Joe Kita
Project Editors Neil Wertheimer, Dolores York
Fact Checking Evelyn Bollert
Copy Editor Barbara Booth
Consulting Art Director Elizabeth Tunnicliffe
Interior Design Vertigo Design LLC
Cover Design Jennifer Tokarski
Illustrations Scotty Reifsnyder
Fitness Illustrations Nicole Kaufman

Reader's Digest **Magazine**
  Global Editor in Chief Peggy Northrop
  Creative Director Robert Newman
  Vice President, General Manager, Reader's Digest Media Marilynn Jacobs
  Executive Editor Tom Prince
  Managing Editor Ann Powell
  Senior Editor Beth Dreher
  General Manager, rd.com Matt Goldenberg
  Assistant Managing Editor Paul Silverman
  Copy Editor Janice K. Bryant
  Editorial Assistant Elizabeth Kelly

READER'S DIGEST BOOKS AND HOME ENTERTAINMENT
President and Publisher Harold Clarke
Associate Publisher Rosanne McManus
Senior Art Director George McKeon
Director, Sales and Marketing Stacey Ashton

THE READER'S DIGEST ASSOCIATION, INC.
President and Chief Executive Officer Robert E. Guth
President, Reader's Digest North America Dan Lagani
President, Reader's Digest International Dawn Zier

FOR VIVAT DIRECT:
Project Editor Penny Craig
Art Editor Conorde Clarke

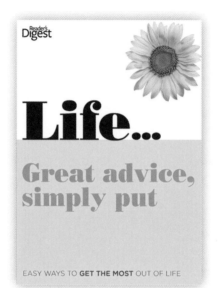

Also Available from Reader's Digest

ISBN 978-1-78020-135-1